WHAT YOU DON'T KNOW
ABOUT HEPATITIS C
CAN HURT YOU!

Who is at risk for hepatitis C? How is it contracted? Who should be tested? ALT, AST, HCV-RNA . . . what do all those tests mean? Are the rumors true?

- Hepatitis C is always fatal: FALSE! While hepatitis C can lead to cirrhosis or cancer of the liver, this is rare. *This book tells you how to manage the disease and avoid its worst consequences.*

- Hepatitis C is primarily acquired from drug use or sexual promiscuity: FALSE! Hepatitis C is more frequently transmitted by infected blood and blood products, and its sufferers come from all walks of life. *Learn how to protect yourself.*

- Kissing and breast-feeding spread HCV: FALSE! Studies indicate that HCV is not transmitted through breast milk or casual contact. *Learn how to protect your loved ones.*

At last! A comprehensive, authoritative book that fights back with *facts* and information that show you exactly what to expect during the course of HCV and exactly what you can do to change the course of the disease for the better. There is hope. There is help. It's all here, in *Living Healthy with Hepatitis C.*

LIVING HEALTHY WITH HEPATITIS C

NATURAL AND CONVENTIONAL APPROACHES TO RECOVER YOUR QUALITY OF LIFE

Harriet A. Washington

Foreword by Steven J. Bock, M.D.

A Lynn Sonberg Book

A Dell Book

Published by
Dell Publishing
a division of
Random House, Inc.
1540 Broadway
New York, New York 10036

Dell books may be purchased for business or promotional use or for special sales. For information please write to: Special Markets Department, Random House, Inc., 1540 Broadway, New York, N.Y. 10036.

Dell® is a registered trademark of Random House, Inc., and the colophon is a trademark of Random House, Inc.

ISBN: 0-440-23608-8

Printed in the United States of America

Published simultaneously in Canada

November 2000

10 9 8 7 6 5 4 3 2 1

OPM

*For Corene Marie Washington
and Percy Cecil Washington,
my parents*

ACKNOWLEDGMENTS

I would like to thank the following experts for generously sharing their expertise and advice or for offering invaluable feedback: Steven J. Bock, M.D.; Robert S. Brown, Jr., M.D.; Yanqui He, O.M.D., L.Ac.; Kenneth Singleton, M.D., M.P.H.; Marcellus A. Walker, M.D., L.Ac.; P. Lounette Humphrey, M.D.; and Michael Carlston, M.D.

I deeply thank the many people with hepatitis C who shared their stories with me in an unselfish effort to improve the lives of other people living in the shadow of the disease.

But most of all I would like to thank my husband, Ron DeBose, for his constant love and support. It makes all the difference.

TABLE OF CONTENTS

If you're looking for authoritative information about hepatitis C, your search is over, because you are holding the very first comprehensive treatment of the subject. As such, it arms the person with hepatitis C with everything he or she needs to face the disease—and win. Within its pages, you will find science and empathy, conventional treatment and alternative therapies, hard facts from physicians and personal stories from those who are struggling with and who have conquered the illness.

Hepatitis C is a health threat that will soon dwarf AIDS in terms of the number of Americans infected. As many as 4 million Americans harbor the hepatitis C virus, but most don't know that they are infected. In fact, it is dubbed the "silent epidemic" because few people experience symptoms to warn them that they are infected.

Clearly, hepatitis C is a serious health threat. You may already know this because newspaper and magazine articles have painted a dire picture of the disease. They have tended to focus upon people who have died or have become incapacitated by hepatitis C. The news media have repeatedly driven home several depressing facts about the disease. There is no vaccine. The only effective medical treatment is expensive, riddled with side effects, and permanently frees only 15 percent of people who try it from the virus.

All this has left Americans with the feeling that the course of the disease is inexorable and fatal and that there is nothing an infected person can do to protect himself or herself.

Fortunately, there are many avenues of hope for this serious disease. But before the publication of this book, relatively few people have been able to read about them. This book explains that hepatitis C progresses very slowly over decades in most people and that its complications kill only a small percentage of infected people. And there is a wide range of treatment options available, which are described in detail. Even if you do not achieve a cure, you can take steps that help you improve the quality of your life and enable you to better cope with the disease.

The message of this book is that hepatitis C is an eminently manageable disease. Its course varies but you can do much to protect yourself from acquiring it, to protect your loved ones from contracting if you are infected, and to protect yourself from its worst consequences.

This book first clarifies the nature of the disease, dispelling the prevalent belief that hepatitis C is usually debilitating or fatal. It then goes on to explain exactly what puts you at risk of the disease and how you can minimize or remove these risks for others.

The book's comprehensive discussion of conventional medical approaches explains in clear detail the virtues and limitations of the chief antiviral drug interferon, alone and in combination as ribavirin. Subsequent chapters explain how conventional medicine can tame acute crises such as liver cancer, mental status changes, and endstage cirrhosis.

But this is only half of the hepatitis C story.

Hepatitis C infection is primarily a chronic ailment, and in this arena, alternative methods offer the type of relief that Western medicine has not. The scientific climate is now expanding to encompass nutrition, herbs, supplements, and nontraditional modalities such as acupuncture. Today organizations such as the

National Institutes of Health acknowledge the important role of diet and lifestyle in management of many chronic ailments.

Accordingly, this work offers chapters on nutritional supplements, herbs, and other natural medicines. They explain how to choose the foods that can best help your liver repair itself and protect against environmental factors that contribute to cirrhosis and cancer. This book shows how food, herbs, supplements, exercise, and other lifestyle changes transform the livers and lives of people infected with hepatitis C. It presents valuable information on cirrhosis and cancer prevention through good nutrition.

As a physician who integrates conventional and complementary medicine to pursue what I have dubbed "progressive medicine" in my own practice, I applaud this holistic approach to the disorder. Many physicians and surgeons, however, are still reluctant to talk about natural approaches to prevention and treatment. But this reluctance shouldn't deter anyone from seeking out and utilizing the most current health information now available. The chapter on conventional treatment explains in detail how to find a physician who is experienced in pursuing complementary treatments.

Equally important, this book explains the important role of the mind-body connection in hepatitis C. It describes many methods that readers can use to harness their mental energy to maximize healing and elevate mood. It offers readers a choice of approaches for dealing with stress and other physiopsychological factors that increase vulnerability to life-threatening complications. Citations from topflight journals such as the *New England Journal of Medicine* and research from institutions such as Harvard and the National Institutes of Health explain the scientific bases for approaches that work.

During the twenty-eight years I have practiced medicine, I have seen in my own practice that a diagnosis of hepatitis C can isolate people with the disease. *Living Healthy with Hepatitis C* banishes this isolation by including the stories of dozens of people with hepatitis C. This book is filled with empathy and it acknowledges the very important psychological component of hepatitis C and its related liver diseases. Written in warm, nonintimidating language, it stresses the positive steps each person can take to recover his or her health. This book has given a voice to scores of people with hepatitis C, who share their personal experiences, challenges, and triumphs.

Melding the best of conventional and complementary medical information, this book offers a cornucopia of information that can help those with hepatitis C regain control over their lives and their health.

Steven J. Bock, M.D.
Director, Center for Progressive Medicine

If you choose to pursue a complementary program for hepatitis C, you must do so under the expert guidance of a qualified physician. In those cases where your physician is unfamiliar with or reluctant to discuss natural treatment methods, you are urged to seek the care and advice of licensed medical experts who practice such adjuvant approaches to treatment.

Hepatitis C: The Manageable Epidemic

Although the world is filled with suffering, it is full also of the overcoming of it.
—*Helen Keller,* Optimism

If you are holding this book because you or someone you love has hepatitis C, you may be deeply frightened.

Don't be.

For a disease that didn't even have a name until ten years ago, hepatitis C has created a lot of anxiety. But the true picture of the disease is not nearly so bleak as it has been painted. There are many steps you can take to help yourself to a long, full life with hepatitis C, or even to a cure. This book is intended as your map on that journey.

The headlines may have already told you that Americans, still reeling from AIDS, are just beginning to realize that we are sitting on an even greater viral time bomb—hepatitis C. The hepatitis C virus, or HCV, can cause serious disease of the liver. The virus enters the body through the blood and attacks the liver, causing it to deteriorate over long periods, as long as ten to forty years. You have read that hepatitis C can cause cirrhosis and liver cancer; in fact, hepatitis C is already responsible for most liver transplants performed in this country. Ten thousand Americans have already died of HCV, and by 2000, more people will die of hepatitis C than will die of AIDS.

Unfortunately, the good news has gotten lost in all the terrifying articles about the "epidemic" of HCV. As opposed to the headline hyperbole, the real challenge of hepatitis C is not dying, but living—well—with the infection. Relatively few people—20 percent—develop life-threatening cirrhosis or liver cancer, the most-feared effects of hepatitis C. And even these can be treated. On the other hand, your chances of permanently ridding yourself of the virus with conventional medications that contain interferon are even lower—15 percent.

This means that if you are infected with the hepatitis C virus, you are *not* likely to die. During a conference on hepatitis C held by the Centers for Disease Control in 1998, Dr. Leonard B. Seef, a senior scientist with the National Institutes of Health, told the *Arizona Republic,* "I would guess that 80 percent of those infected are going to outlive their disease." He compiled a report demonstrating that fewer than half of patients with hepatitis C had significant liver disease, even twenty-four years after they were diagnosed with hepatitis C.

But until better treatments are developed, you are not likely to be cured, either. You are most likely to develop a chronic, very slowly progressing condition that you can learn to manage. You will have to contend with symptoms that can range from annoying to energy-sapping, but most of these problems are controllable if you understand the disorder and if you know what to do. Many of the disease's complications can be delayed, made milder, or even prevented by using the suggestions in this book.

Most people with hepatitis C can manage their condition with a combination of early diagnosis, timely medical treatment, and lifestyle changes.

The odds are heavily in your favor, so promise yourself that you will not become paralyzed by fear. Instead, become prepared. The difference between being incapacitated by pain and fear and living fully is, like so many things in life, a matter of knowledge and preparation.

Picking up this book is the first step in the right direction. This book will demystify everything about hepatitis C. It will show you how to decipher the alphabet soup of laboratory test results and tell you what does and does not put your friends, coworkers, and loved ones at risk for contracting the virus. This book will tell you exactly what to expect during the course of the illness and exactly what you can do to change the course of the infection for the better. From this one book, you will learn about both cutting-edge conventional medicine for hepatitis C and about natural approaches that help you to live well with the disease.

You probably have a lot of questions, such as: *How did I get HCV? What symptoms will I develop? When? Will I get worse? How quickly? How can I avoid infecting others? What do my test results mean? What treatments are available? Which should I choose? How can I maximize my chances of a cure? Failing that, how can I stay as healthy as possible? What alternative treatments work? What if I need a liver transplant?* You may have already discovered that finding reliable answers is not easy.

This book will answer all these questions and many others. It offers you a scientifically accurate and detailed explanation of what medicine has to offer you—in plain, jargon-free English. This book also stresses the critical importance of recruiting a physician to be your health advocate. It tells you exactly how to select the best-qualified physician and other health-care providers.

But this volume offers you even more. It differs fundamentally from other books for people with hepatitis C in its unprecedented completeness. This book fills the large treatment vacuum left by conventional medical treatment by explaining what complementary therapies have to offer. It doesn't tell you only about blood tests, interferon, and liver transplants or only about diet, herbal approaches, and acupuncture. This book covers both conventional and alternative medical approaches for you in clear, easily understood language with a few uncomplicated tables and charts. In its pages you will find:

CUTTING-EDGE CONVENTIONAL INFORMATION. Interferon, the only effective conventional medication for hepatitis C, can retard liver damage but cures only about 15 percent of the people who try it. It is expensive and carries significant side effects such as fatigue and depression. This book offers up-to-the-minute information about conventional medical treatments, including daily interferon regimens, combination therapies such as pegylated interferon and ribavirin, protease inhibitors, genetic approaches, and partial-organ liver transplants. These phrases may be Greek to you now, but after reading Chapter 4 you will understand them all, as well as all your options for conventional hepatitis C treatment. Chapter 4 also describes treatments on the horizon, one of which may turn out to be the long-sought "magic bullet" that allows a more efficient cure.

ALTERNATIVES THAT WORK. Meanwhile, herbs, supplements, acupuncture, and other remedies can help alleviate the worst symptoms of hepatitis, such as fatigue, depression, swelling, pain, and other physical discomforts. Diet and nutrition, including supplements, are also very important in treating that key digestive organ, your liver. Rigorous medical studies suggest that some of these remedies can also address the underlying disease process, bolster the immune system, retard liver damage, and help to restore your blood-test values to within normal limits.

This book will tell you what works and what doesn't, with references to many controlled, peer-reviewed clinical studies in such publications as the *Journal of the American Medical Association, Gastroenterology,* and the *New England Journal of Medicine*. It will also show you how to evaluate the credentials of alternative practitioners and tell you which groups can direct you to practitioners whom you can trust. This book also offers a selection of treatment plans that have worked for others and that you and your doctor can tailor to your needs. These incorporate a conventional medical approach with a variety of self-help and complementary medicine regimens.

THE MENTAL DIMENSION. You are more than a liver. In fact, you are more than just a body. The emotional, mental, and spiritual component of your fight against hepatitis C infection is equally important, and so this book approaches the person with hepatitis as a whole person with a spectrum of emotions triggered by the illness. This book illuminates the complex connections between hepatitis C, anger, and depression. More important, it tells you how to go about finding emotional and spiritual support that allows you to confront and conquer fear and anger. It gives practical advice on using exercise and a whole armamentarium of alternative therapies such as acupuncture, guided imagery, and prayer to reduce the stress and depression that so often accompany this disease.

Living with hepatitis C can be a lonely affair. Few people understand the disease, so it tends to be stereotyped as a "junkie's disease." (Many people simply don't realize that many infected people acquired the virus during blood transfusions or other medical procedures.) Support groups are an important remedy for this sense of misunderstanding and isolation. Such groups offer you emotional support, as well as tips for educating your loved ones.

The chapters of this book are also enriched by personal vignettes from people who are living with hepatitis C. More than forty people with hepatitis C generously shared their experiences, frustrations, and triumphs with me, and I have shared some of these with you. Their stories illustrate how they have confronted and dealt with some of the very symptoms and uncertainties that you can expect to face during the course of your illness.

Before you go on to the detailed answers in this book, see "What This Book Covers" on page 8. It offers you a quick overview of the book's contents. But first, here is some succinct background information on the rise of hepatitis C, to help you understand what you are up against.

The Rise of Hepatitis C

Hepatitis C, or HCV, has long been a shadowy entity. It caused disease for decades before scientists even named it. They knew that a form of hepatitis that was neither hepatitis A nor hepatitis B existed. They called it, logically enough, non-A, non-B hepatitis. Hepatitis C was identified in 1989 and a blood-screening test followed quickly in 1990, but not before HCV had widely infiltrated the blood supply. Many people were infected by blood transfusions before 1990, but the transfusion risk was almost completely eliminated by 1992.

Even today, people commonly confuse hepatitis C with the other forms of hepatitis, such as A, which can be caused by contaminated food, or B, which can be transmitted sexually. Even spouses and close friends may fear touching or eating with a person with HCV. This means that one of your challenges will be educating your friends and family about the disease and reassuring them that you can protect them from the risk of contracting hepatitis. This book will give you all the information you need to be able to ease their minds.

Between 28,000 and 180,000 people are infected with hepatitis C each year, according to the Centers for Disease Control and Prevention, or CDC. Many don't discover their infection until signs of liver failure appear decades later. This has prompted some to call hepatitis C the "silent epidemic." Use of the term *epidemic* is controversial, but whatever you call it, there is no question that 3.9 million Americans are chronically infected with the hepatitis C virus, and few of them know it. Four times as many people have hepatitis C as AIDS, but unlike AIDS, hepatitis C is not usually fatal.

People do die of hepatitis C, however, especially if they are not diagnosed until extensive, irreversible liver damage has set in. In the year 2000, more people will die of HCV than AIDS, and deaths will reach 30,000 by 2020. However, after that, the deaths will level off because blood screening has all but eliminated the risk from transfusions. Increased public awareness of HCV risks should lower the numbers of infected people, too. As people come to understand that drug use, piercing, and tattooing put them at risk, fewer people will engage in these behaviors.

Today, one of every fifty Americans has the hepatitis C virus, but most have no idea that they are infected, or how they acquired it.

Some groups are even more hard-hit, including medical workers, hemophiliacs, the poor, minorities, and drug users, even one-time "experimenters." Health and hospital workers are at a four-times-higher risk than the general public because they are more frequently exposed to infected blood. Nearly all adult hemophiliacs, who rely upon infusions of blood products to live, were infected before the blood supply was first screened in 1990.

As many as one of every ten young black men is infected, a shocking statistic that is only the tip of the iceberg for African Americans. Black Americans are not only at higher risk for hepatitis C, they are also less likely to be helped by interferon. Social, economic, and medical factors conspire to make minority-group members less likely to receive a liver transplant if they need one. All this means that it is especially important for African Americans to understand hepatitis C and to learn how to maximize their chances of getting first-rate medical care.

Like HIV, hepatitis C is spread in infected blood. But because widespread screening now protects the blood supply, hepatitis C is usually transmitted today by controllable behaviors such as drug use or tattooing.

There are other parallels to AIDS as well. Many people at high risk have not been tested and so don't know they are infected; and the virus went undetected in the blood supply, leading to many infections through transfusion.

One of the most troubling parallels to AIDS is that, as you will see in Chapter 2, the U.S. government has failed to follow through on its responsibility to warn people who are at risk. Just as the government faltered in warning Americans about an HIV-contaminated blood supply in the early day of the AIDS epidemic, the government has failed to honor repeated commitments to warn everyone who may have received HCV-tainted blood or blood products before 1992.

But there is an important difference between HIV and HCV: HCV is usually not fatal. It is important for you to understand this, because the word *virus* causes many people to react by feeling that they are doomed or tainted. What's more, the news reports often focus upon the most dramatic cases—people who are deathly ill or dying. The focus of this book is where it belongs for people with hepatitis C—on life.

What This Book Covers

In this book you will find everything you need to know to take control of your health. Each chapter concludes with a list of references for further reading and resources where you can find the help and treatments it describes.

CHAPTER 1: THE NATURAL HISTORY OF HEPATITIS C. This chapter opens by describing how a healthy liver functions. Then it clearly explains what the hepatitis C virus is and how it causes illness. It also demystifies the alphabet soup of hepatitis A, B, C, D, and E, and explains how they differ. The chapter continues with a broad overview of the disease's natural history, from the initial symptomless infection to serious conditions such as cirrhosis and liver cancer.

CHAPTER 2: TRACKING THE RISKS OF HEPATITIS C. This chapter gives you detailed information on how to control the risk of infection. It details exactly what is and isn't risky behavior, exactly how to protect your spouse, family, and friends from the virus—and how to reassure them that it is safe to be close to you.

CHAPTER 3: GETTING A DIAGNOSIS. Hepatitis C is called "silent" because only one in four people experiences early symptoms, and many of these are so mild that they do not lead people to their doctor's office for tests. People with HCV tend to be diagnosed by accident when a routine blood test reveals the disease. This is a serious problem because early diagnosis is key to getting the most effective treatment and to making the lifestyle changes that can limit your liver damage. This chapter explains who should be tested. For those who have been diagnosed with HCV and who face a lifetime of laboratory tests as part of monitoring their health, this chapter translates the arcane language of laboratory tests into plain English for you.

CHAPTER 4: CONVENTIONAL TREATMENT: CURE FOR A FORTUNATE FEW. Chapter 4 explains exactly how to find the best hepatitis C expert for you, an alternatives-savvy doctor who will become your partner in healing and your advocate within the medical system. Next, it explains how interferon works, as well as its costs in money, side effects, and relapses. Finally, this chapter offers up-to-the-minute information about other conventional medical treatments, including combinations of interferon and other medications, genetic approaches, and treatments that are still being tested.

CHAPTER 5: FOOD: DIETARY ARMOR FOR YOUR IMMUNE SYSTEM. Good nutrition is an essential part of your strategy for living well with hepatitis C, and conventional and complementary practitioners alike acknowledge nutrition's key role in health and recovery. Nutrition is especially important in promoting liver health because the liver is the body's nutrient warehouse. This chapter will explain how the right foods in the right forms ease the biological stress on this hardworking organ, and how the right nutrients enhance the action of the immune system, which is fighting the HCV virus and its effects.

CHAPTER 6: DIETARY SUPPLEMENTS. This chapter focuses upon the most solidly promising nutritional and other supplements in the treatment of hepatitis C. They cannot cure the disease, but case-controlled clinical studies offer evidence that many do the next best thing by bolstering the immune system and retarding or preventing liver inflammation and damage.

CHAPTER 7: HERBS. Fortunately there are herbs that help to improve the overall health and well-being of people with hepatitis C. Some also restore liver blood tests back to normal ranges, an indication that liver damage has stopped progressing. This chapter offers background information on the range of herbal treatment modalities. It then details the use of specific herbs for a natural approach to living with hepatitis C. It describes each herb's actions, recommended manner of administration, and specific dosages.

CHAPTER 8: TAMING THE LIVER'S ANGER. The emotional component of liver diseases such as hepatitis C has been recognized for centuries and verified by contemporary medical doctors, who repeatedly observe that depression is a common feature of the illness. To counter the emotional devastation of hepatitis C, this chapter details lifestyle choices such as drug and alcohol avoidance and exercise. It also describes how prayer, acupuncture, psychotherapy, and guided imagery can help you tap your inner resources to alleviate the emotional upheaval of hepatitis C. Last but definitely not least, it will show you how to find a support group and how to reach out to the huge multifaceted network of experts and your fellow travelers with hepatitis C.

CHAPTER 9: PUTTING IT ALL TOGETHER. This chapter lays out the basic philosophy and elements of the HCV treatment plan. It will detail the main components of treatment plans incorporating herbal support, a dietary strategy, and nutritional supplementation as a blueprint for you to tailor to your situation under the guidance of your doctor. This chapter will also describe successful strategies adopted by practitioners to help people with HCV escape serious illness.

CHAPTER 10: EXTREME REMEDIES: LIVER TRANSPLANTS AND EXPERIMENTAL TREATMENT FOR ADVANCED DISEASE. Complementary approaches to serious HCV illness can maximize the body's natural ability to resist liver failure and serious symptoms such as crippling fatigue and nausea. But people who develop the serious complications of endstage cirrhosis and liver cancer need aggressive Western medical treatments such as liver chemotherapy, radiation, and surgery, including liver transplantation. In fact, HCV infection is already the biggest cause of liver transplants, and a fierce competition for scarce livers already exists. The information in this chapter will help you to plan ahead to maximize your chances in the unlikely event that you will need a liver transplant. It also provides information about organizations and research centers that may be able to help, as well as newer techniques such as partial-liver transplants.

CHAPTER 11: HEALING RESOURCES. This chapter tells you exactly where and how to find the best written resources, natural practitioners, advocacy organizations, and Web sites. It also provides specific addresses, phone numbers, and Web site addresses.

My intent in writing this book has been to provide you with a trusted guide as you learn how to live with and manage hepatitis C. I hope it will help you to understand that you are not helpless and that you are not alone.

For more information

The following articles may be of interest:

Brown, David. "Girding for an 'Emerging' Illness: Current Treatment for Hepatitis C Doesn't Work Well—But Ongoing Research Offers Hope." *The Washington Post,* September 22, 1997.

Chase, Marilyn. "Hepatitis C Epidemic Lurks in the Afflicted as Blood Tracing Lags." *The Wall Street Journal,* October 19, 1998.

Groopman, Jerome. "The Shadow Epidemic." *The New Yorker,* May 11, 1998.

CHAPTER ONE

The Natural History of Hepatitis C

There is no darkness but ignorance.
    —*William Shakespeare,* Twelfth Night

Knowledge is your first priority in learning to treat your hepatitis C. You should understand how a healthy liver functions so that you can better understand exactly how the hepatitis C virus threatens your health. As we have seen in the Introduction, the virus infects the liver, causing chronic disease in most infected people and causing extensive cirrhosis or liver cancer in a minority. This chapter will explain how a healthy liver functions. It will then give you a detailed description of the hepatitis C virus and how it can impede the smooth functioning of this hardworking, versatile organ.

Structure of the Normal Liver

Your liver is a three-pound marvel. It is the largest organ in your body, arguably the most hardworking, and easily the most versatile. Your liver is also the only organ in your body that regenerates itself, even if three quarters of it has been destroyed by disease or poisoning. But you need a functioning liver in order to survive, so once the liver is harmed beyond its ability to recover or survive, death is imminent.

The liver purifies and disarms toxins and plays key roles in the synthesis, breakdown, and activation of important biological molecules. What's more, your liver is an important part of both the digestive and the immune systems. The liver is often compared to a filter, but it is more akin to a chemical factory complex with many functions that are key to your survival.

If you've ever seen a beef liver in the supermarket, you have a good idea of what your own liver looks like. It is shiny, smooth, reddish brown, and roughly triangular. It lies tucked under your ribs, with the largest portion on your right side and a smaller lobe on the left. Your liver is surrounded by other vital tissues and organs, including the kidneys, diaphragm, lungs, intestine, and colon.

The liver is fed by two major blood vessels. The *hepatic artery* carries bright red oxygen-laden blood from the lungs to the liver via the *abdominal aorta*. The *hepatic vein* takes dark red deoxygenated blood (blood from which the oxygen has been depleted)

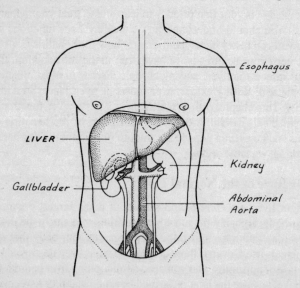

Esophagus

LIVER

Kidney

Gallbladder

Abdominal Aorta

Figure 1: *The liver*

from the liver back to the heart. The liver's largest source of blood is the *portal vein,* which delivers blood from the digestive organs and the spleen. Tiny branches of the hepatic artery and the portal vein deliver nutrients and oxygen, and carry away poisons and manufactured chemicals. The dark red blood that suffuses this network of tiny blood vessels in the liver gives the organ its dark-reddish hue.

Between the microscopic blood vessels there are specialized liver cells that transport, store, and process fats and other substances in the liver. These include *Kupffer cells,* which are the "incinerators" of the liver. They absorb the detritus of metabolic wastes, unwanted toxic chemicals, and microbes. These cells then use their internal enzymes to break down and neutralize these dangerous substances.

Liver tissues are comprised of tiny spherical components only one fifth of an inch across, called *lobules.* Lobules in turn are made of sheets of cubical cells called *hepatocytes* that are nourished by nutrients in the blood. Each hepatocyte in this network manufactures bile, a detergent substance that is necessary for fat digestion. Each hepatocyte delivers bile to its area of the liver matrix as well as to the gallbladder, the small adjacent organ that stores bile.

When you eat a piece of salmon or another fatty food, bile flows to the liver through the *common bile duct,* which passes through the liver, gallbladder, pancreas, and intestines.

The Liver's Major Functions

The liver's major functions include purification, metabolism, and synthesis.

PURIFICATION.   The liver rids the body of literally hundreds of chemical pollutants and drugs. All the blood in your body passes through the liver, and as it does, the liver filters and detoxifies it. The liver neutralizes all sorts of dangerous toxins, from noxious dry-cleaning and gasoline fumes to nicotine, alcohol, prescription medications, and illicit "recreational" drugs.

The liver also absorbs poisonous substances from the intestine, and transforms them into innocuous ones that it releases into the bile, which is excreted from the body. The liver also inactivates toxins produced internally, such as the poisonous compound ammonia. Ammonia is a by-product of protein metabolism that the liver converts to *urea*, which can be safely excreted in urine.

METABOLISM. The liver breaks down or converts many substances from molecules that would harm the body into substances that the body can use for fuel or to build tissue. For example, the liver also metabolizes alcohol, changing it from a metabolic poison into harmless components that are excreted in urine. The liver also breaks down excess cholesterol. Cholesterol has gotten a lot of bad press, but some cholesterol is necessary for bodily processes such as making collagen. However, too much cholesterol clogs the arteries, leading to heart attack and stroke. Cholesterol also deranges body chemistry in more subtle ways; for instance, the most common type of gallstones contains excess cholesterol. The liver prevents excessive cholesterol by moving excess cholesterol into the bile, whence it is stored in the gallbladder, then eliminated from the body.

SYNTHESIS. *Synthesis* in this sense means the construction of biological materials. The liver builds important biological molecules and tissues. For example, the liver employs amino acids as chemical building blocks to build several types of proteins. (It also uses amino acids to make fuel for the body's energy production.) The special proteins that the liver makes have important functions: These proteins enable your blood to clot, carry nutrients, and even regulate hormone levels. These proteins also control the complex balance of chemicals and fluids in your body. For example, the protein *albumin* regulates the amount of various bodily fluids, including the volume of plasma in your blood.

The liver also forms, or synthesizes:

- **Blood.** Before birth, the liver forms all types of blood cells— *red blood cells,* which carry oxygen, *white blood cells,* which participate in immune-system defense, and *platelets,* which are cell fragments used in blood clotting. The liver regulates plasma, the liquid component of blood. Liver diseases such as hepatitis C affect all of these blood components.

- **Bile.** We've already seen that the liver makes bile. This brownish green fluid contains cholesterol, water, sodium, potassium, chloride, proteins, and bilirubin. Bile digests many substances, especially fats and the fat-soluble vitamins A, D, E, and K. The liver uses bile to transform oily substances that are insoluble in water into water-soluble substances that can be carried in the bile. Bile is stored in the gallbladder and released as needed to metabolize fat.

- **Lymph.** The healthy liver filters enough plasma from the blood to generate about a liter of *lymph*. Lymph is a fluid that carries proteins, sodium, potassium, and other minerals through the body. The flow of lymph follows conduits that are analogous to blood vessels. They run from the liver to lymph channels in the abdomen. From the abdomen, lymph is absorbed into the bloodstream. But hepatitis C upsets the regulation of lymph flow.

This sounds like enough work for any one organ, but the formation of blood, bile, and other important bodily fluids is merely the tip of the iceberg when it comes to the many varied responsibilities of the liver. This versatile organ carries out many other key functions, including:

NUTRITION. Your liver is the body's nutritional workhorse. This important digestive organ produces the bile that allows proper processing of fats and also metabolizes the protein and carbohydrates that provide energy for the body's maintenance and activities.

NUTRIENT STORAGE. The liver is a nutrient warehouse that maintains large stores of fat, sugars, vitamins, iron, and other nutrients, sending them out to "fill orders" from parts of your body that need energy or nutrients.

DIGESTION. The liver governs the digestion of fats. It produces bile and chemically related bile acids, which absorb fats through the lining of the small bowel and ferry them into the bloodstream. The bile acids are then reabsorbed in the small intestine and recycled into the liver, to be used again. Extra fat is stored in the liver and elsewhere. Your liver releases these stored fats to supply alternate fuel when your body runs out of carbohydrates.

Complex carbohydrates such as bread or pasta must be broken down into the sugar *glucose* before your body can use them for energy. The liver stores glucose as *glycogen*. Later, when your body needs energy, the liver turns glycogen back into glucose, transporting it through the blood to satisfy the body's needs.

ELIMINATION. The liver processes waste products and discharges them in the urine. It eliminates neutralized poisons into the bile, and they are excreted as solid waste in the stool. In fact, components of bile give normal stool its brown color.

REGULATION. The multitalented liver is a key regulator of many important chemicals in the body. In order to regulate their levels, the liver activates and inactivates some hormones and drugs. It regulates the amount of blood components and plasma levels. Besides balancing blood-sugar levels by releasing glycogen when needed and managing the transport of fat through the body, the liver helps regulate hormones. For example, it balances the amount of male sex hormones such as testosterone and female sex hormones such as estrogen in the blood.

IMMUNE SYSTEM. The immune system is a fascinatingly complex biochemical defense system, and the liver is an integral part of it. All sorts of infection-fighting white cells, including fibroblasts, lymphocytes, macrophages, and plasma cells, are made in the liver. It's not necessary to learn the special roles of all these white cells; just remember that the immune system and the liver are closely dependent upon each other.

Now that you know the many important functions of the healthy liver, we can address the central question, *What is hepatitis C and how does it damage the liver?*

The Hepatitis C Virus

The term *hepatitis* simply means inflammation of the liver. Hepatitis can be caused by anything that damages the liver, such as poisoning. More than one hundred drugs are known to poison the liver. So, too, are common commercial chemicals such as the industrial solvent toluene, carbon tetrachloride, as well as trichloroethylene and vinyl chloride, which are used in dry cleaning. The yellow phosphorus used in some rat poisons causes hepatitis, as do several very poisonous mushrooms, notably *Amanita*. Hepatitis is sometimes caused by bacterial infection and by many viruses, including herpes, rabies, HIV, and influenza.

But hepatitis is also caused by certain viruses that specifically target the liver, and hepatitis C is such a virus. Hepatitis C is a *viral hepatitis*.

A virus is big trouble in a small package. Incredibly tiny even on the microscopic scale, a virus is visible only with the aid of an electron microscope. And no wonder: A virus is no more than a single molecule of DNA or RNA wrapped in a protein coat. DNA (deoxyribonucleic acid) and RNA (ribonucleic acid) are the genetic molecules that constitute the blueprint for an organism's heredity and design. RNA and DNA are called the molecules of life, but a virus is not a truly living organism. A virus is an invisible parasite that cannot perform any living functions or reproduce itself until it infects a host cell.

Viruses invade the living cell, in this case a liver cell, and hijack the machinery the cell uses to propagate itself. The virus causes the cell's RNA or DNA to make more virus instead of liver cells. Then the millions of copies of virus cells burst from the host cell, killing it. Each new virus infects another host cell to make even more copies. Viruses can spread quickly.

The hepatitis C virus, or HCV, is an RNA virus. It is of a type called a *flavivirus* and resembles the viruses that cause yellow fever and dengue fever. There are six genetically different variants of HCV, called *genotypes,* categorized by the type of enzymes they need to reproduce. As we will see in Chapter 4, "Conventional Treatment," these genotypes have significance for the treatment of hepatitis C.

Through most of the 1980s, the medical literature referred to "non-A, non-B" (or NANB) hepatitis, so dubbed by scientists who realized that many people with hepatitis didn't have hepatitis A or B. Scientists knew that hepatitis A and B could be transmitted by blood transfusions and had been screening donated blood for A and B since the 1970s. But increasing numbers of people were becoming infected by NANB hepatitis. In 1989, the Centers for Disease Control identified a separate virus that was responsible for almost all NANB hepatitis, which it dubbed hepatitis C. A screening test for the HCV virus was developed later that year and was refined a few years later.

At first, medical experts were ecstatic. Now people could be routinely tested for hepatitis C. Blood donors could be screened to make sure they were not carrying the virus, and existing stores of donated blood could be tested for the virus. But soon epidemiologists—scientists who study disease patterns in groups—were appalled to discover that the U.S. blood supply was already heavily tainted with the newly discovered virus. (Now, as you will read in Chapter 2, the blood supply is safe.)

Private physicians became equally worried when it became clear that relatively few people were being tested for HCV. They were worried because so many of those who were tested—one in fifty—harbored the virus. In some groups, such as young African-American men, the rate was much higher, as many as one in ten. The rate of HCV infection has slowed, but as Chapter 2 explains, many people still do not know they are infected.

There is still a lot of confusion surrounding hepatitis C in the minds of the public. Besides hepatitis A, B, and C, there are hepatitis D, E, F, and (possibly) G viruses, and a few other candidates are still being studied. People with hepatitis often find that their friends, family, and coworkers confuse these strains. For example, they may shrug off your announcement that you are infected because they think you have contracted hepatitis B, which most people can fight off successfully even without treatment. Or they may think that you have contracted hepatitis A, and warn you to observe better hygiene and be careful what you eat, because HAV is caused by fecal contamination and is often foodborne. For easy reference, check the "Types of Hepatitis" table on page 22, which compares and contrasts the most important characteristics of the known hepatitis viruses.

Another sign of confusion is that people with HCV must often fight the stigma of hepatitis C as a "drug addict's disease." Drug addicts *are* at high risk for hepatitis, but HCV is also spread by blood and blood products. This means that working in a hospital, tattooing, piercing, blood transfusions, kidney dialysis, and a host of other blood-sharing activities also place you at risk. Chapter 2 explains the risks of acquiring HCV—and how to avoid them—in great detail.

So much for what HCV is not: What *does* happen if you are infected?

Acute Infection

In traditional Chinese medicine, the liver is called the "battleground of the body." War is a good metaphor for what happens when HCV attacks. When the virus enters your bloodstream, it targets your liver. The virus particles invade your liver cells and viral RNA hijacks the cell's reproductive machinery, forcing the liver cells to produce more virus. Your immune system perceives this takeover and sends antibodies and lymphocytes to stop the virus production. This is the *acute* phase of hepatitis C.

The body goes into emergency mode, pulling out all the immunological stops to halt the invader. Unfortunately, in the end your liver is suffering damage via a dual attack—from the virus and from your own overzealous immune system. Your immune system launches a counterattack that is florid but inefficient,

Types of Hepatitis

TYPE	TRANSMISSION	SYMPTOMS	NATURAL HISTORY	TREATMENT	VACCINE	BLOOD SCREEN?
A	water or food tainted with human waste, or direct contact	nausea, jaundice, pain, darkened urine, light stools appear within a month	spontaneous recovery within 6 months; confers immunity	no conventional treatment; herbs and dietary treatments can ease symptoms	yes	yes
B	sexual contact, blood and other bodily fluids, shared needles	fatigue, malaise, jaundice	92–98 % recover spontaneously; others become carriers	interferon alpha 2-b; lamivudine; famcyclovir; Chinese herbal treatments improve liver enzyme levels	yes	yes

C	blood-to-blood contact	mild or none for 10–40 years	15 % recover spontaneously; 85 % develop chronic illness; 15 % of chronically ill cured by interferon; 5–20 % of chronically ill require liver transplants	interferon, alone or with ribavirin; herbal treatment lowers liver enzyme levels; supplements support the liver and immune system	no	yes
D	can infect only people with hepatitis B; bloodborne and sexual transmission	worsens hepatitis B	95 % recover spontaneously	treatment that cures hepatitis B also cures D; interferon alpha 2-b; Chinese herbs	B vaccine prevents infection with D	blood tests detect D only sporadically

(continued)

Types of Hepatitis continued

TYPE	TRANSMISSION	SYMPTOMS	NATURAL HISTORY	TREATMENT	VACCINE	BLOOD SCREEN?
E	food and water tainted with human waste; most cases from developing countries	immediate; nausea, jaundice, pain, darkened urine, light stools	spontaneous recovery within 6 months	no conventional treatment	offers only limited protection	no
F	not well characterized; most experts now think F does not exist	no consensus exists	chronic, with liver failure	no conventional treatment	no	no
G, also called GB virus	bloodborne; but some researchers now doubt that hepatitis G exists	unclear; acute, chronic, and fulminant hepatitis	chronic hepatitis in 70–85 % of infected adults	no conventional treatment	no	yes, but it is unreliable

damaging the tissues of the liver. This immunological defense usually fails to stop the virus.

In fact, most of the actual damage to your liver is caused by "friendly fire" from your own immune system, not direct damage by the virus. Specialized infection-fighting proteins called *antibodies* latch on to the virus and try to deactivate it. They do this by fitting themselves to an *antigen* on the surface of the virus—just like a key fitting into a lock. Then the white cells move in to destroy and absorb the virus-infected cells. But it is hard for antibodies to get a good grip. The hepatitis C virus is particularly good at eluding the immune system. It mutates rapidly, shifting its shape to prevent antibodies from latching on to it. In the end, antibodies usually succeed only in inflaming and destroying parts of the liver itself.

As this battle for control of the liver progresses between the virus and the immune system, the infected person may sense that something is amiss. He or she may experience a few days of fever, inflammation, muscle aches, chills, and a stiff neck. But these early symptoms of infection are so mild that many people never notice them at all. Because these symptoms are brief and resemble the flu, those who do experience them are apt to dismiss them as harbingers of a minor illness.

Brief, mild symptoms or no symptoms at all make hepatitis C an insidious illness. Because there are so few symptoms, very few people seek medical help and very few are diagnosed with hepatitis C during this early, or *acute,* phase of the illness. This is unfortunate, because during this period, the amount of virus in the body, or the *viral load,* is very low. As Chapter 4 explains in detail, recent research suggests that treatment is most successful in people with low viral loads. If more people with hepatitis C were diagnosed during the earlier stages, more would be cured and more would escape serious illness.

For about 15 percent of HCV-infected people, this early battle between the virus and their immune system ends in victory. They rout the virus from their bodies during this acute phase, they do not become ill, and they do not spread the infection to others. If they are given tests for HCV infection, the tests reveal that they were once infected and now are not. This is the best possible outcome of an HCV infection.

Chronic Infection/Inflammation

The other 85 percent of people infected by the HCV virus develop *chronic* infection, or an infection that persists. The infection creates inflammation, or hepatitis, so they are said to have chronic hepatitis. (Technically, a chronic infection lasts more than six months, but most chronic hepatitis C infections are lifelong.)

As we have seen, lymphocytes attack the virus-infected cells by releasing chemicals that usually damage and kill the liver cells without stopping the virus. This damage continues, but the liver has many extra cells and it can regenerate, growing new ones. As a result, the damaged liver can still carry out its

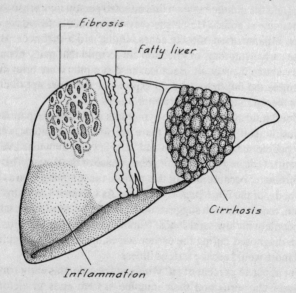

Figure 2: *Drawing of a diseased liver, exhibiting areas of inflammation, fibrosis, fatty liver, and cirrhosis*

many functions, and the infected person experiences only mild symptoms for a very long time. Most people have very mild or no symptoms during the first ten years or so of hepatitis C. Many experience some degree of fatigue and a few people eventually develop jaundice, a yellowish discoloration of the skin and eyes. Even fewer people develop mental problems such as trouble concentrating. Fewer still experience a sudden, dramatic liver failure, called *fulminant hepatitis*. Fulminant hepatitis is very rare.

Despite the lack or dearth of symptoms, the infected person can spread HCV to others via blood and blood products, so he or she is an *asymptomatic carrier*.

Fibrosis

Fibrosis is the next stage of liver damage. Fibrosis is a condition that arises when dead liver cells harden into nonfunctioning scar tissue on the liver. This is a result of years of fighting the infection. After a decade, the livers of most HCV-infected people show significant areas of fibrosis. But because there are so many extra liver cells to take over the activities of the dead cells, even large injured sections of the liver can lose function without any overall diminution in liver function.

For 66 percent of people with chronic hepatitis C, liver damage never progresses beyond this stage, and their health is not seriously compromised because their livers still function. As we saw in the Introduction, relatively few infected people progress to the next stage of liver disease, even after twenty-five years. Clearly, all the newspaper and magazine articles that predict dire fates for everyone with hepatitis C are wrong. They paint a uniformly bleak picture that is not supported by the facts.

Cirrhosis

Unfortunately, for 33 percent of the people with chronic hepatitis C, the damage worsens. The liver's capacity for regenerating new healthy tissue is not infinite, and *cirrhosis* of the liver results if the fibrosis eventually extends enough to seriously distort the structure and function of the liver. When we hear the word *cirrhosis,* we automatically think of alcohol abuse, but cirrhosis can be caused by many things. The liver can be assaulted by disease, nicotine, fried foods, medications, alcohol, and illicit drugs. It is a pretty hardy organ and can usually handle this abuse in small, infrequent doses. But over many years, the hard-working liver often pays the price for our indulgences. Years of inactivating these and other poisons on a daily basis can injure liver tissues, causing cirrhosis.

What does cirrhosis mean? Blood and lymph can no longer flow readily through the cirrhotic liver. The liver's many functions fail, causing a domino effect of serious symptoms and deficiencies throughout the body.

Among these are:

JAUNDICE. The cirrhotic liver cannot excrete bilirubin, the yellowish pigment in bile. The bilirubin pigment accumulates, giving a yellowish cast to the whites of the eyes and to the skin.

ESOPHAGEAL VARICES. These are blood vessels in the esophagus that rupture and hemorrhage very easily, resulting in uncontrolled bleeding from the mouth. This bleeding is terrifying and very dangerous. Esophageal varices are due to liver damage that impedes the blood flow through the liver's scarred portal vein and hepatic artery. The backed-up blood is diverted through other veins and arteries, including those in the esophagus. But these blood vessels were not designed to handle the pressure of this extra blood flow, so they break and bleed easily.

ASCITES. Hepatitis C can cause lymph to collect and pool in the abdomen, resulting in a abdominal swelling called *ascites.* When the pooling of lymph causes swelling in the legs, it is called *edema.*

ENCEPHALOPATHY. We saw earlier that the liver is responsible for neutralizing ammonia, a toxic by-product of protein metabolism, then excreting it from the body. But a badly injured liver cannot process ammonia, so it builds up. This ammonia poisons the brain and causes mental changes such as confusion and, in extreme cases, even coma.

UNCONTROLLED BLEEDING. The cirrhotic liver can no longer make specialized proteins, including *prothrombin,* which is necessary for blood clotting. This means that a person with cirrhosis can bleed easily, even from minor bumps or scratches.

PORTAL HYPERTENSION. Have you ever watered your lawn with a garden hose? If you squeeze the hose tightly enough, the water will back up, causing a ballooning of the hose behind your thumb. This is akin to what happens to the blood flow from your spleen through the portal vein to your liver. The scarring in your liver decreases blood flow the same way your thumb decreases water flow though a garden hose. The backup of blood flow in your spleen creates pressure, just as the water backup forces the walls of the garden hose to balloon out. This resulting pressure is called *portal hypertension.* The backup of blood places pressure on the other internal organs, including the spleen, where many blood cells are stored.

CRYOGLOBULINEMIA. A damaged liver can begin producing damaged proteins, a condition called *cryoglobulinemia.* A host of distorted blood proteins can cause nervous-system and kidney damage. Cryoglobulinemia also causes severe, persistent itching. Itching can also be caused by morphine-like toxins that the liver can no longer clear from the body. This itching can be as difficult as pain to live with, and it is not helped by over-the-counter lotions or creams. Fortunately, it can be treated with prescription medications.

OSTEOPOROSIS. Liver dysfunction results in too few bone-building cells, which can make bones brittle. Adding calcium or vitamin D doesn't help, because the cirrhotic liver cannot always absorb and process them properly.

KIDNEY DAMAGE. Hepatitis C can put you at risk for kidney diseases as well. A disorder with the tongue-twisting name *membranoproliferative glomerulonephritis* is the most common kidney disease associated with HCV infection. Others include *membranous glomerulopathy, fibrillary glomerulonephritis, rapidly progressive glomerulonephritis,* and *IgA nephropathy*.

APPETITE LOSS, WEIGHT LOSS, MALNUTRITION. A badly damaged liver cannot metabolize fats or fat-soluble vitamins. This leads to nausea whenever you eat foods with fat in them. An extensively cirrhotic liver may not be able to break down stored fats. Streaks of stored fat are visible on the liver, causing the condition called "fatty liver," which is common among alcoholics whose livers are damaged. Alternatively, the fat may be excreted in stool where it is visible as whitish bands and called *steatorrhea*. Cirrhosis affects many aspects of nutrition. For details, see Chapters 5 and 6.

THYROID DISEASE. Because the liver helps regulate thyroid hormones, thyroid problems are common in people with hepatitis C. For details about hepatitis C and thyroid disease, see Chapter 4.

Like hepatitis C itself, cirrhosis is insidious because laboratory tests may be normal in someone with the early stages of cirrhosis. And some people with cirrhosis have no symptoms at all. As I explain at length in Chapter 3, it is very important to have regular examinations and monitoring tests by your physician. This is the only way to catch cirrhosis at its earliest stages, before extensive damage has set in. This is also when your treatment options are greatest.

Endstage Cirrhosis

After twenty or more years with HCV infection, some people enter its final stage, called *endstage cirrhosis*. The liver has become so extensively scarred and has lost so much function that liver failure is inevitable. You cannot live without a functioning liver, because no other organ can perform its many essential roles. Among the many symptoms that afflict people with endstage cirrhosis are jaundice, ascites, easy bruising, wasting (loss of muscle and fatty tissues), bleeding varices, encephalopathy, and incapacitating fatigue. People who develop liver failure need transplantation, the only effective treatment today for endstage cirrhosis. A liver transplant can cure most people with endstage cirrhosis. As you will see in Chapter 10, liver transplantation is a transforming experience that gives jaundiced, sickly, weak, frightened people with cirrhosis their old energy and vibrant lives back.

Fortunately, fewer than one in ten people with chronic hepatitis C suffers such extensive cirrhosis.

Liver Cancer

About 5 percent of people with hepatitis C develop liver cancer, although some estimates place the rate slightly higher, at 10 percent. People with liver cancer also need liver transplants. But only people with a few small cancerous tumors are good candidates for liver transplantation. People with many tumors or large tumors are more likely to have cancer that has spread to other organs, and a liver transplant cannot cure these cancers. So again, it is very important to have your health regularly monitored by your physician. If you are one of the unfortunate few people to develop liver cancer as result of hepatitis C, you want to catch it when it is small, localized, and treatable. See Chapter 10 for more about the diagnosis and treatment of liver cancer.

Transplants transform the lives of people with endstage cirrhosis or liver cancer, but sadly, there are too few organs to go around. Some people die waiting for an organ. But, as you will read in Chapter 10, there are steps you can take to maximize your chances of obtaining a successful liver transplant.

Now that you understand the basic nature of hepatitis C and how it affects your health, it is time to address other important questions: *How can you minimize the risks of hepatitis C? How can you avoid contracting hepatitis C, and if you are infected, how can you protect others?* Chapter 2 will tell you.

For more information

National Digestive Diseases Information Clearinghouse
2 Information Way
Bethesda, MD 20892-3570
(301) 654-3810
Provides basic facts about hepatitis C.

Centers for Disease Control and Prevention (CDC)
Hepatitis Branch, Mailstop G37
National Center for Infectious Diseases
Centers for Disease Control and Prevention
Atlanta, GA 30333
CDC Public Inquiries: (800) 311-3435
CDC Hepatitis Hotline: (404) 332-4555. This hotline permits you to automatically request information that will be faxed to your machine.

NIAID Office of Communications
National Institute of Allergy and Infectious Diseases (NIAID)
Building 31, Room 7A50
Bethesda, MD 20892
(301) 496-5717
Provides fact sheets and other information that is also available on the NIAID home page: www.niaid.nih.gov/.

"Hepatitis A, B, and C: Questions and Answers"
gopher://gopher.uiuc.edu/oo/UI/CSF/health/heainfo/diseases/
contag/hepa
A brief page describing the differences between various types of hepatitis, with information on prevention and treatment.

The home page for the National Institutes for Health, www.nih.gov/, also directs you to information on hepatitis.

Public Health Department

Call your county or state Department of Public Health for information about hepatitis C educational resources in your area.

CHAPTER TWO

Tracking the Risks of Hepatitis C

Chance favors the prepared mind.
—Louis Pasteur

I had a blood test a few years ago and it showed that the hepatitis C antibody was present. But I don't have a clue when I got sick!

Susan

For the most part, my family has been supportive, but they tend to be a little judgmental. They hear "hepatitis C" and picture you with a needle in your neck. And you know what, even IV drug users don't deserve this.

Mary

Hepatitis C is not just an individual disease. The virus infects an individual, but the accompanying fear that infects his or her partner, family, and community can be just as devastating. When people hear that HCV is a bloodborne virus, they are likely to think of AIDS and to be afraid that they will catch a fatal disease from you. But as you now know, HCV is rarely fatal. Like AIDS, it is *not* spread by casual contact. Unlike AIDS, it is *not* usually spread sexually between partners.

The All-American Virus

If you are infected with HCV, you have plenty of company: One of every fifty Americans has the hepatitis C virus. Groups that have been particularly hard-hit include medical workers, hemophiliacs, the poor, and minorities. Drug users are at high risk; not only habitual users, but also one-time "experimenters."

But despite the stereotypes, the risk is not concentrated in groups that have suffered societal discrimination, as has happened with gay men and, later, minority-group members who contracted AIDS. HCV sufferers are the guy next door, with a good job, mortgage, and 2.3 kids. Perhaps he experimented with drugs once or twice in college. Perhaps he encountered the virus while a soldier in the sexual revolution of the 1970s. Perhaps he had his ear pierced in a dubious establishment twenty years ago. Maybe he acquired HCV while saving lives in an ambulance. Maybe he has no known risk factors at all.

We can't point to a physically distinct group and say, "They are at risk; I am not." But we can change our behaviors, and to protect ourselves and our loved ones, we must learn behaviors that can minimize our risks and the risks of spreading hepatitis C to others.

Hepatitis C can be a lonely disease. Many people, even those who love you, may fear closeness because they are afraid of catching hepatitis C. The irony is that the risk of acquiring a new case is now lower than it has been in many years. What's more, HCV is hard to catch unless you share blood. It is easy to protect those whom you love from infection once you learn how. That is the purpose of this chapter. When you have read it, you will understand what puts a person at risk for HCV. You will understand how you or someone you love may have contracted it. And you will understand how to protect your family and regain intimacy without fear.

You probably have many questions: *How did I become infected? Can I infect my husband or wife? My children? Is it safe to kiss, hug, or eat with an infected person? Is HCV spread by coughing or sneezing? By sharing a can of soda? Can I become infected by living with an infected person? If I'm infected, can I safely bear children? Breastfeed? Can a person get HCV from a blood transfusion? From an organ transplant? From drugs? From drinking? From a prostitute?* This chapter will answer them all.

Experts cannot explain how everyone acquired the virus, but most people will better understand how they may have been exposed after they understand the many ways in which one can contract it.

This chapter will also explain in detail what is *not* risky, and why scientists have determined that certain activities and factors are safe. You must also understand this, too, so that you can reassure the people you love, work with, and meet. Happily, people's worst fears about catching the disease are unfounded. A family can safely share a home without fear. Couples can safely kiss, hug, and share intimacy.

Blood: The Key to Risk

HCV is a bloodborne virus, which means it must use blood or a blood component to travel from one person to another. In that sense it is hard to become infected: You have to actively inject infected blood into your body.

The U.S. blood supply became contaminated with hepatitis C in the 1970s and 1980s. Epidemiologists think that injected-drug users were largely responsible for the spread of the virus through the blood supply. They sold or donated blood that was later transfused, infecting others, some of whom later donated *their* blood. Soon our blood supply was awash in HCV and no one knew. Half a world away, soldiers of the Vietnam War were often exposed to medical procedures such as transfusion and vaccinations under nonsterile conditions in the field and brought HCV back from the war with them. The rise of a new disease, AIDS, created an additional pool of people whose immune systems made them vulnerable to infections, including HCV.

Epidemiologists think that it took only a few years to extensively infect the blood supply. Then people who had acquired HCV via transfusions spread the virus through drug use, tattooing and piercings, and certain types of sexual practices.

But kissing, hugging, eating with your family or roommates, sharing the newspapers and remote control, talking, laughing, tickling your children, dancing—all the shared pleasures of friendship and love—do not involve sharing blood, so they do not put you at risk for HCV.

You cannot spread HCV to family members or spouses by sharing a household, from using the same bathroom, the same furniture, phone, appliances, linens, and dishes, or by breathing the same air or coughing or sneezing. In the past there was some academic confusion about risk because studies show that a family with one chronically infected person is slightly more likely than other families to have another member develop an infection. But a report in the *Annals of Internal Medicine,* and most subsequent U.S. studies, suggest that this is because each family member was independently exposed to a source of infection, not because one family member infected another. Perhaps, for example, both family members are hemophiliacs, work in hospitals, had tainted transfusions, or got tattoos at the same unsanitary establishment.

Yet it *is* possible to spread HCV and infect a family member if you share blood. To avoid this risk, family members should not:

- share razors, needles, manicure scissors, clippers, or any other sharp implement that can draw blood.
- share toothbrushes.
- touch the blood or wound of someone with HCV.
- be careless with used sanitary products. Menstrual blood can transmit the virus, so be especially careful to wrap and carefully discard used sanitary products. Common courtesy and hygiene would dictate this anyway.

Mosquitoes and other biting insects do not transmit HCV. Experts theorize that this is because the virus does not replicate in the body of the mosquito, so it cannot complete its life cycle and infect others.

Transfusions: A Legacy of Risk

Before 1990, one in every ten people who received a life-giving blood transfusion also received an unwelcome guest: the hepatitis C virus. The National Institutes of Health (NIH) estimates that 90 percent of the hepatitis acquired through transfusions is due to HCV. By 1992, 1 million Americans had received blood and blood products from donors who subsequently tested positive for hepatitis C. The federal government now recommends that everyone who received a blood transfusion before 1992 be tested for HCV.

Every mode of transmission is not equal. Becoming infected through a transfusion is an especially efficient way to get HCV directly into the bloodstream. People who are infected by a direct injection of tainted blood into their veins include people who had transfusions, hemophiliacs, and long-term IV drug users. They tend to have more of the virus in their bloodstreams and are more likely to suffer medical problems such as liver failure.

The good news is that transfusions rarely transmit the virus today, thanks to improved screening procedures that detect HCV antibodies. As you probably remember from Chapter 1, antibodies are produced by your immune system to attack the invading virus. Their presence constitutes indirect evidence—"fingerprints"—of the virus. The first blood screening test for HCV antibodies was introduced in 1990, and a more precise test, the EIA, in 1992.

So today there is very little risk of acquiring hepatitis C from a blood transfusion. The NIH estimates that only 3 of every 10,000 blood recipients contract HCV. In fact, not one of 650 transfused people in an ongoing NIH study has acquired HCV from receiving blood.

Circle of Contagion

Now that an accurate test protects the blood supply, what puts you at risk for hepatitis C today? Today's risk factors have to do with introducing infected blood directly into the body.

These risk factors fall into one of two categories: The first is *avoidable risks*. These are risks that you can easily avoid, such as illicit drug use, tattooing and piercing with improperly cleaned needles, and sex with multiple partners. The second category consists of *unavoidable risks* that you typically cannot avoid, such as dialysis and contaminated organ transplants.

Avoidable Risk Factors

The most important avoidable risk factors include drug use and body art (tattooing and piercing). By avoiding the risk factors detailed below, you can minimize your risks of acquiring HCV.

> I'm pretty sure I contracted the virus during the six or seven years that I was an IV drug user. I also have a couple tattoos, and had unprotected sex with multiple partners for many years. I could have caught the disease from any of the above, but specialists have pretty much narrowed it down to the needle use. I started using drugs and alcohol at age fifteen and didn't stop until I was thirty-four years old and had lost custody of my children. Fortunately, I was court-ordered for every possible evaluation, put on monitored Antabuse therapy, and decided I had to fight for those kids. It took three long years, but I did it! They are now twenty-five, eighteen, twelve, and eight . . . and all carry scars from the past, but we are together as a family and all have had lots of therapy. . . . I've been clean for seven years and would like to add that I am one of the fortunate people who got out of the madness of drugs and alcohol successfully. . . . Many don't make it.
>
> Sage

DRUGS. Thinking about the health hazards of drug use tends to summon up the stereotyped hollow-eyed, homeless, long-term addict whose arms are scarred with needle tracks. But drug-acquired HCV also threatens the middle-aged suburban executive who has never touched a needle. You don't have to be an addict or even a frequent user of drugs to court risk: One or two instances of injecting drugs can infect you, because injecting the drug places the virus directly into the bloodstream with horrible efficiency. Studies suggest that it takes fewer viral particles to infect one with HCV than with HIV, so a single episode of drug use is more likely to result in hepatitis than in AIDS.

In fact, many people with HCV acquired it from a single, long-forgotten episode of "experimentation" with injected drugs, as much as twenty years earlier. However, long-term drug users are more likely to become infected than single-time experimenters.

Flushing a needle with cleaning solution may not kill all the virus, and the virus may persist even if no blood can be seen. Unfortunately, we don't have to worry just about fresh blood. HCV can survive outside the body for extended periods of time, even in dried blood, infecting another person up to three months later.

This leads to yet another drug hazard: sniffing cocaine. Studies have repeatedly found "a very strong association with intra-nasal cocaine use." Here's why: Snorting cocaine irritates the lining of the nose, leaving the interior of the nostrils raw and bloody. It can even erode the septum, the middle section of cartilage between your nostrils. The straw or rolled-up paper used to sniff cocaine picks up blood from the nostrils. When it is used by another person, even weeks or months later, he or she is exposed to whatever was in the first person's blood. Because it came from a drug abuser, it is likely to be tainted with HCV.

If you have a substance-abuse problem, you must tame it in order to avoid HCV. Don't try to go it alone. Discuss it with your doctor and ask him or her to refer you to experts for help. See Chapter 11 for information about organizations that can help you.

By the way, nicotine is another drug associated with HCV. Smokers have a slightly increased HCV risk, probably because smoking undermines immune-system function. So HCV provides another reason to stop smoking,

BODY ART. Tattoos were once the province of sailors, cycle gangs, and self-proclaimed rebels, but now they've gone mainstream. The skyrocketing popularity of tattooing and body piercing may promote another wave of infection; they are already responsible for 2 percent of HCV infections. Tattoo artists use needles to drive colored ink into the skin, creating permanent designs. As we've seen, the virus survives in dried blood, so if these needles are not *scrupulously* cleaned after every use, they can transmit viruses.

Body piercing has become more popular, too, including multiple piercings in sites other than the earlobe. If needles are reused without being thoroughly cleaned, the same risks apply. To avoid them, have body art performed where only disposable needles are used and thrown away after each use. Failing that, needles should be sterilized at high temperatures. Avoid piercing sites such as the septum of the nose and the cartilage of the upper ear, because, unlike the earlobe, they are not well supplied with blood and the body cannot get infection-fighting white blood cells to the site.

Some cosmetic procedures carry the same risks as tattooing. "Permanent" eyeliner is a form of tattooing that can spread disease if the needles are not scrupulously sterilized. So can electrolysis. Be sure to ask a cosmetologist to use a new needle before placing yourself in his or her hands. If you're not convinced that the needle is sterile, don't risk it.

NONMONOGAMOUS SEX. Ten percent of people with HCV reported having had sexual contact with an infected person. But when it comes to HCV, all sexual contact is not equal. Monogamous sex is safer than sex with multiple partners.

So often, though, hepatitis C drives an unnecessary wedge of fear between husbands and wives. They fear physical contact, especially sexual intercourse. This robs the couple of intimacy and deprives the infected person of an important source of comfort and support. Hugging and kissing carry no risks of exposure. But for sexual intercourse between long-term monogamous partners, the picture is less clear.

After a confusing period when the medical studies seemed to contradict each other, scientists now realize that the risk of transmitting HCV to a faithful long-term partner, even if you have sex frequently, is low. The American Liver Foundation estimates it at less than 1 percent. "I can't recall ever having seen a case," adds Dr. Adrian di Bisceglie, medical director of the ALF.

The CDC places the HCV risk of a longtime monogamous partner higher—as high as 5 percent. But this risk may have little to do with transmission via sexual intercourse. According to a 1994 study in the *Annals of Internal Medicine,* the partners of infected people who acquired HCV had independent risk factors that could account for their infection. This means that they may have acquired the virus because they both had body art with tainted needles or both had invasive health-care procedures from an infected practitioner or both used drugs.

Older partners of a person with hepatitis C are slightly more likely to acquire it, due to the natural weakening of the immune system with age.

Condom use reduces the risk of transmission, but no long-term studies have quantified this. The Surgeon General's office calls the sexual risk so low that couples in long-term relationships do not need condoms, but until scientists can definitively determine how much of this risk is due to sexual transmission, monogamous couples *should* use a condom.

The CDC recommends that spouses or long-term sexual partners of newly diagnosed patients be tested for HCV. A good way to allay the fears of a spouse is to suggest he or she take the test, which will probably be negative. Then the doctor should take that opportunity to explain how low the risk is and to suggest using a latex condom.

If either of you is infected with HIV or herpes, this increases the chance you will transmit HCV to your partner, so condom use becomes even more important. Avoid anal sex, which is more likely to result in small tears in the rectum through which hepatitis C could enter. You should also avoid sexual contact while menstruating, because of the possible exposure to blood.

Just as living with an infected family member is safe, living with a spouse will not endanger you if you observe a few commonsense precautions. In a nutshell, avoid contact with blood. Don't share a razor or even a toothbrush, which can harbor trace amounts of blood.

On the other hand, people who have multiple sex partners do have a higher risk of contracting HCV. A *Journal of Infectious Diseases* study found that risk factors associated with transmission to the sexual partner included more than twenty-four lifetime sexual partners and sex with a commercial sex worker, that is, a prostitute.

These elevated risks reflect a game of sexual roulette—the more sexual partners one has, the more likely one is to encounter an infected person. People with multiple partners are also likely to suffer from the sexually transmitted diseases that make it easier for HCV and other viruses to gain entry through lesions, rashes, pustules, and other breaks in the skin. A study of patients in a clinic for sexually transmitted diseases (STDs) found that their infection rate was much higher than that of the general population. As many as one in five people treated in STD clinics may harbor the virus. People with many sexual partners are also more likely to be commercial sex workers who are at higher risk for drug use, assault, forcible rape, and other dangers that expose them to blood and increase their HCV risks.

A 1994 *Journal of Infectious Diseases* study of 309 couples being treated for STDs suggests that it is easier for men to infect women with HCV than for women to infect men with the virus.

Heterosexual or homosexual people share the same risks of contracting HCV, with the important caveat that active or passive anal sex significantly increases one's risks, as just mentioned.

The best thing about avoiding all the risk factors detailed in this chapter is that by doing so you will be protecting not just your liver, but your overall health.

By avoiding drugs you avoid addiction, death by overdose, HIV infection, STDs, stroke and neural damage, and a host of serious psychiatric problems, including the risk of suicide—to say nothing of serious social problems such as losing your children, spouse, job, and home. Sexual contact with multiple partners is never a healthy move anyway, because it increases the risks of AIDS and so many other STDs. If you stop smoking, you lower your risks of cancer, heart disease, stroke, and a Pandora's box of other illnesses.

Other HCV Facts You Should Know

IT'S SAFE TO BREASTFEED.   CDC studies show that breast-fed babies are no more likely than others to contract HCV. Because nursing protects against many infections, physicians do not discourage it.

KISSING.   The NIH says kissing is safe because HCV inhabits saliva in very small amounts, but no definitive studies have established this. Human bites can transmit HCV, however.

DON'T DONATE.   It's probably clear by now that you should not donate blood if you are infected with HCV. Don't donate semen or eggs, either. If you donate an organ or part of an organ, the recipient will acquire HCV, but as you will see on page 49, this is sometimes an acceptable risk.

VACATION RISKS.   In some countries, HCV control is feeble or nonexistent, so you must be aware of the risks of medical treatment abroad when traveling for pleasure. See also "Foreign Birth and Travel" on page 51.

Unavoidable Risk Factors

You can't avoid everything that puts you at risk for HCV. You can't change your ethnicity, gender, or whether you received a lifesaving transfusion before 1992. Poverty and socioeconomic status are hard to change, and even those who propel themselves to better environments and economic brackets find that many medical risks have already affected them.

But there is value in knowing what unavoidable risks you face. Forewarned is forearmed. If you know that your medical history or ethnicity puts you at risk, you can use that knowledge to minimize your risk.

First, if you have any of the risk factors described in this chapter, get tested, if you haven't been already. Next, realize that your higher risk means you should be especially vigilant of seemingly innocuous symptoms like unexplained fatigue or flulike symptoms.

If any of the unavoidable risk factors pertains to you, it is especially important that you bolster your immune system in every way possible, because a healthy vigorous immune system is your body's first defense against a viral attacker. Chapters 5 through 8 will show you how, in detail.

HEMOPHILIACS. We have seen that blood transfusions are now safe. But *hemophiliacs,* whose blood doesn't clot well, need highly concentrated blood products called *factors,* made of blood products from hundreds of people. Without clotting factors, hemophiliacs risk life-threatening internal bleeding. Using blood from so many people multiplies a hemophiliac's chance of receiving infected blood to a near certainty. Today hemophiliacs can use artificial factors without HCV risk, but for an entire generation, the damage has been done. Almost all adult hemophiliacs are infected.

CHILDREN. Children can acquire hepatitis C in three ways: Estimates vary widely, but as many as one in twenty newborns has antibodies to HCV and *may* have been infected by his or her mother during birth. Other children received HCV from tainted blood transfusions before 1992. Still others received contaminated intravenous immunoglobulin therapy such as Gammagard before 1992. Mercifully, the disease is milder in children.

FROM MOTHER TO CHILD. It is very unlikely that a U.S. mother will transmit HCV to her unborn children; it is more likely that the baby will acquire the mother's antibodies to HCV during birth, which does not mean that the baby has HCV.

Although blood tests and the usual assays will detect these anti-bodies and so may give positive results, the babies are not chronically infected with the virus itself.

In a Japanese study, 6 percent of infants born to women with hepatitis C were infected with HCV. But no long-term U.S. studies have yet quantified the risk of passing hepatitis C to your baby; this will take time. As a matter of policy, pregnant women are not now tested for HCV because the costs of screening would be high and we don't know how to prevent the rare cases of mother-to-child transmission. However, you should have an HCV test if you are planning to become pregnant, so that you will know whether your baby will face this risk, however small. Treatments may become available to lower the small risk of transmission and you will not be able to take advantage of them unless you know your baby is at risk.

AGE. The immune system begins to weaken by the thirties, so the number of HCV-infected people peaks between the ages of thirty and fifty.

Occupational Hazards

I'm a health-care worker who was infected at work. I worked with surgeons. It's ironic that I've taken care of ill people my whole life. I try to use the little energy I have on a daily basis to do positive things But when I think of the people they *know* are infected and are not telling . . . !

Albert, a nurse

I'm a forty-six-year-old single mother of four, and I was diagnosed just two months ago. I believe I probably contracted the virus in 1978 while working as a lab assistant in a hospital. But it doesn't really matter how, I just wish the public was better informed about the disease and that everyone knew that *anyone* can have it. I'm struggling with the stigma that it's a "junkie" disease, and the ignorance of some that it's highly contagious. My four children are hep C free, and we have not practiced any precautions for sixteen years.

I'm active in the YMCA, a certified EMT and a social worker, and have been in recovery [AA] for over three years. Things have been great. Now, my future is uncertain.

Madhu

HEALTH-CARE WORKERS.   Many health-care workers cannot avoid being exposed to their patients' blood. Gloves and eye shields afford only limited protection. Most at risk are phlebotomists, who draw blood for a living, doctors (especially surgeons and emergency-medicine specialists), and nurses, especially those who work in emergency departments and trauma centers. Tell any health-care worker who treats you that you have HCV so that he or she can take precautions.

Medical risk is a two-way street. Doctors, surgeons and obstetricians have transmitted HCV to patients during procedures. No laws currently bar HCV-infected professionals from operating unless and until they infect a patient.

EMERGENCY MEDICAL TECHNICIANS AND FIREFIGHTERS are also at risk, because they are exposed to the blood of the accident victims they treat. They are often exposed to blood when they give mouth-to-mouth resuscitation. Performing emergency invasive procedures such as starting IVs and giving injections in the field is also risky.

POLICE OFFICERS face similar risks from disaster and crime victims.

LABORATORY TECHNICIANS and even **NONMEDICAL HOSPITAL WORKERS** even are also at risk for infection via needle sticks and exposure to patient blood. There are rules and procedures to minimize risks, but they don't always work.

I had bagged the trash in the research laboratories. I was always very careful to wear gloves. As I lifted a bulging plastic bag into the large bin, it bumped against my leg and I felt a sharp pain; it was a needle. Doctors and technicians know that they are supposed to put all needles into the sharps bin, but someone didn't. I walked right over to the emergency department, shaking all the way. They gave me gamma globulin and some other medications, but said they could not figure out what was in the needle that stuck me. I'm really scared, because this was a research lab: I could have been injected with anything! What if it was something they have no treatment for? Every time I get a sore throat or a headache, I worry.

Rose

Military Service

I had an airborne accident on August 29, 1976, where another jumper and I became entangled. We were jumping around fifteen hundred feet. They say I bounced two times when I hit the ground. I broke both legs, my back, my hip and my lung collapsed. I had two operations and two transfusions. About a week or so after the surgery my eyes turned a little yellow and I was put in quarantine. They said, "It's nothing." Just a year ago, I tried to give blood and discovered that it *was* something: hepatitis C.

David, a veteran

Like emergency medical personnel, soldiers are exposed to higher risk factors for HCV. They may come into contact with infected blood during their combat training or when receiving vaccinations, transfusions, or medical treatment. This is especially true if they serve abroad in regions with high rates of infection, such as Asia and North Africa. If they are treated locally for emergencies, they run the risk of unscreened transfusions and injections from improperly cleaned needles. Conditions in the field are often nonsterile. In some regions acupuncture needles are not cleaned properly before reuse and disposable hypodermic needles are not available.

In November 1997 researcher Gary Roselle published the first large study of hepatitis C infection in Veterans Administration (VA) patients. This survey documented a steady climb in the number of antibody-positive patients, and the actual number is probably much higher, because most veterans are not treated in VA medical facilities.

YEAR	NUMBER OF CASES	PERCENT INCREASE
1991	6,612	——
1992	8,365	21%
1993	14,097	213%
1994	18,854	285%

Roselle suggests that Vietnam-era veterans, now in their forties and fifties, are at much greater risk of infection than the rest of the population, due to the large numbers of transfusions given under primitive conditions during the Vietnam War. But the Department of Defense (DOD) disagrees. It has cited other studies that find no evidence that military members are at greater risk. The Board of Veterans Appeals says it cannot show sufficient evidence of a connection between veterans' military service and their hepatitis C disease. This is bad news for veterans, because it means fewer benefits for hepatitis C treatment.

Medical Procedures

DIALYSIS.   A kidney dialysis machine takes over a failing kidney's function, cleansing the blood. But inadequately cleaned machines put patients at a high HCV risk. In a Tufts University study of dialysis patients who had not received transfusions, 16 percent had antibodies to HCV.

ORGAN TRANSPLANTS.   These fall into the "unavoidable risk" category because a person on a waiting list for a transplant needs a new kidney, liver, or heart to live and so has no choice. Every potential organ donor is tested before the organ is used, so doctors know if an organ is contaminated. But there are times when receiving an organ that is infected with hepatitis C makes sense, for example, if the recipient already has hepatitis C.

Even if the recipient is not already HCV-infected, he or she will die shortly without the organ, so if there are no well-matched, uninfected organs available, it is worth the risk. The liver damage may not progress, and if it does, it is treatable. For many transplant recipients, exchanging a long-term risk for imminent death is a good bargain.

Institutionalization

Crowded conditions such as are found in jails, psychiatric hospitals, and homeless shelters foster the spread of HCV, as they do many infectious diseases. There are no exact nationwide statistics, but 1994 studies by the state of California found that 41 percent of male and female prisoners were infected with hepatitis C. Many public-health experts think that this mirrors the national prevalence in the penal system. In prisons, the increased risk is also due to the higher incidence of drug use, tattooing, and violent acts in which blood is spilled, including anal rape.

Poor people and minorities are more likely to have been incarcerated or institutionalized; this may account for some of their higher risk.

Poverty

HCV is not an equal-opportunity infection. A 1992 *New England Journal of Medicine* report revealed that the frequency of HCV antibodies stood at 18 percent—ten times higher than the national average—among people in an inner-city Baltimore emergency room.

There are many poverty-associated risk factors. Poor people enjoy less-continuous, lower-quality medical care. They are more likely to live in crowded circumstances, and more likely to suffer from the STDs that serve as "gateway infections" to HCV. Poor people don't use drugs more often than wealthier ones, but they do have higher rates of injected drug abuse, which means that the average poor person is more likely to have intimate, possibly blood-related, contact with a drug abuser.

Ethnicity

So many people in my community don't understand or don't know what hepatitis C is and have no idea that they are at such high risk. No one has told them that they can be sick and feel fine. They're worrying about avoiding AIDS and treating hypertension with no clue that something else could be killing them right now. I'm from New York City, and we are known for being loud and aggressive, so I guess it's on me to bring the message home: If you had a blood transfusion from before 1992, go get tested. You could have chronic hepatitis; I do.

Erika

According to the American Liver Foundation (ALF), African Americans have the highest infection rate for hepatitis C: 3.2 percent of African Americans and 2 percent of Hispanics are affected, in comparison to 1.2 percent of Caucasians. African-American men have a startlingly high rate—one in ten of all thirty- to forty-nine-year-olds, the highest risk group. This high infection rate contributes to the high death rate of black males.

Foreign Birth and Travel

If you were born in, have lived in, or have visited countries where HCV is more prevalent than in the United States, you may already have been exposed to a higher HCV risk that you cannot control. Travel can also be an occupational hazard: It is mandatory for people in military and diplomatic service. Journalists and other employees who are "offered" overseas assignments often find they have few alternatives to travel.

Infection control is less meticulous in many countries. For example, a December 1998 study by the World Health Organization found that of twelve South American countries surveyed, not one screened its blood supply for HCV. Also, more virulent strains of HCV abound abroad.

While you are abroad, avoid invasive medical treatment such as transfusions, shots, and IVs whenever possible. One of the best ways to do this is to safeguard your health before you leave home. Make sure you are vaccinated against all diseases you may encounter; don't confine yourself to those vaccinations the law requires. Also, learn something about health practices in lands you are visiting. You should make sure you know where the best facilities are when visiting a country where sterile procedures are difficult to pursue and blood testing is sporadic or absent.

You can easily obtain information about the HCV risk in countries you have visited by calling your local health department, the CDC, or a voluntary organization such as Healthcare Abroad and The International Association for Medical Assistance to Travellers. Their addresses and phone numbers are given at the end of this chapter.

HIV Co-Infection

Two of every five people with HCV also have HIV. In doctors' lingo they are *co-infected*. Doctors used to consider the HCV infection a long-term issue and HIV infection a medical emergency, so they focused upon the HIV infection in co-infected people. But two major developments during the past few years have made AIDS experts reevaluate the significance of co-infection. Firstly, cutting-edge HIV treatment such as protease inhibitors are now allowing people with HIV to live longer lives. Co-infected patients have begun surviving long enough to succumb to liver disease, with their HIV under control. Secondly, patients whose livers have been damaged by HCV often cannot take protease inhibitors because of their toxicity. This robs them of years of health.

Now experts know that co-infection accelerates liver damage alarmingly, and makes it harder for people with HIV to stave off AIDS as well. Remember the mention of genotypes in Chapter 1? Co-infected people with genotype 1a are at special risk: They progress to AIDS much more quickly than those with other genotypes.

To summarize, people who are at elevated risk of hepatitis C include:

- People who received blood or blood products before 1992
- Hemophiliacs
- African Americans, especially men
- Health-care workers and laboratory technicians
- The institutionalized, including people in prison
- Vietnam-era veterans
- Emergency medical technicians, firefighters, and police officers
- Drugs users/experimenters
- People who have undergone dialysis
- People who have received invasive medical care abroad
- Hispanics/Latinos
- People who have HIV or an STD
- People who have had multiple sexual partners, especially prostitutes
- The poor

But for 40 percent of people with HCV, we don't know what put them at risk. Some of these people may have been exposed to forgotten or unrecognized risks such as having had a medical procedure abroad. Medical papers often suggest that some of this "mystery risk" is attributable to youthful drug use that people deny because they don't realize that snorting cocaine could have put them at risk. But this seems unfair. Because 40 percent is such a large figure, HCV experts think that there are important risk factors that we don't know about.

People with HCV often say they are frustrated to find themselves stereotyped as drug users. On March 5, 1998, Ann Jesse, executive director of the Hepatitis C Connection, testified before a congressional subcommittee that it took twenty years for her infection, acquired during a blood transfusion in 1973, to be diagnosed. This was due to "the perception of my doctors that a sixty-two-year-old Caucasian grandmother didn't fit the usual profile of a patient."

Carroll M. Leevy, Sr., M.D., director of the Sammy Davis Jr. Liver Institute in Newark, New Jersey, told the same committee that 30 percent of his patients from suburban New Jersey who were coming in for treatment were without any identifiable risk factor for the disease.

Fateful Intersections

More people with HCV have contracted the virus from medical procedures than from illicit drugs, and they understandably resent being stereotyped as drug users. Stereotyping the HCV-infected person as a drug addict is also cruel because it implies that an addict is somehow less a victim, and less worthy of care and concern. Not only is this untrue, the distinction is scientifically false, because it reinforces a popular fallacy that the world can be divided into high-risk and low-risk groups.

There are many unexpected intersections between people we think of as "high risk" and others. The HCV in the hemophiliac's blood factor may have come from a prostitute. The prostitute herself may have been infected by a surgeon whose occupation put him at risk. A good example of such an unexpected intersection is the Canadian connection. Last year, Canadians were outraged to learn that a private U.S. firm shipped HCV-infected plasma from Arkansas prison inmates north when U.S. regulations forbade its use in the States. Thousands of "low-risk" Canadians have been infected.

Without Warning

We've been amply warned about AIDS, SIDS, Lyme disease, and toxic shock syndrome, though none of these affects nearly as many people as HCV. There are warning labels on wine bottles, cigarette packages, and even on ladders. Where are the health warnings for HCV?

Unfortunately, the government has not yet warned the people who are most at risk. One million Americans who acquired HCV from the nation's blood supply have no idea that the transfusions that saved their lives also put them at risk.

"IT'S IN THE MAIL." For almost eight years, the government has been promising to look back through medical files, then send warning letters to everyone who received a blood transfusion before 1990. The letter would explain that they are at risk for hepatitis C and should be tested. Surgeon General David Satcher repeated the promise of a nationwide "lookback" program in October of 1998. But most of our mailboxes are still empty. Some individual cities have sent letters, but this is a drop in the proverbial bucket.

As a result, many people are walking around with untreated HCV. They are possibly infecting others and certainly risking liver damage that could have been arrested if they had known the truth years ago. There are also holes in our understanding of HCV that might be filled if all exposed people were tested. We also cannot know how prevalent the infection really is or completely understand its risk factors.

In a positive development, the Surgeon General's office revealed in mid-1999 its plans to warn people about the risks of hepatitis C via mass-media announcements.

If and when the government does widely acknowledge that Americans were infected by a contaminated blood supply, there could be financial consequences. The Canadian government illustrated this in early 1999, when it established a $1.1 billion fund to compensate Canadians infected with hepatitis C through the blood system. The estimated 6,500 Canadians infected from 1986 until 1990 are to receive an initial payment of at least $10,000 plus additional compensation of up to $220,000 depending on the severity of the illness.

This chapter has detailed HCV risks for you with clear, readable explanations. This will enable you to discard your needless fears, and take necessary action to protect against the real risks. With this information you will be also able to reassure your friends and loved ones. But this book is no substitute for the care of a licensed physician. It is critically important to see your physician regularly and to rely upon his or her advice. Medical information changes quickly, and general data and recommendations may not apply to you. Therefore, your doctor's advice should supersede anything you read here or elsewhere.

For more information

Bibliography

You may find these publications about the risks of hepatitis C of interest:

Chase, Marilyn. "Hepatitis C Epidemic Lurks in the Afflicted as Blood Tracing Lags." *The Wall Street Journal,* October 19, 1998.

Groopman, Jerome. "The Shadow Epidemic." *The New Yorker,* May 11, 1998.

Organizations

For help in avoiding infectious risks abroad, contact:

Healthcare Abroad
243 Church Street West
Vienna, VA 22180
(800) 237-6615; (703) 281-9500
Publishes *Health Guide for Travellers*.

The International Association for Medical Assistance to Travellers
417 Center Street
Lewiston, NY 14092
(716) 754-4883

International SOS Assistance
P.O. Box 11568
Philadelphia, PA 19116
Within PA: (215) 244-1500
Outside PA: (800) 523-8930

Online sources

The HEP Education Project

This nonprofit organization distributes educational materials and information about support groups through the Web at www.scn.org/health/hepatitis/. Share these publications with your family and friends.

HCV Activist Mailing List

Concerned about government inaction around hepatitis risks? This list focuses on political action to promote HCV research and funding. It works through coordinated letter writing and other group efforts. To subscribe, type in the body of the e-mail message "SUBSCRIBE HCV ACTIVIST" and send the message to: majordomo@statsrus.com.

CHAPTER THREE

Getting a Diagnosis

When I moved to New York, I just wanted my new doctor to sign the form that would allow me to use the company gym. But he insisted on doing a physical, So I came in, not with a very good attitude because I felt tired and I was getting the flu to boot.

When I told him I had muscle soreness and a slight fever and was really tired from the stress of moving, he began asking me all sorts of questions about my medical history. I told him that I was healthy as a horse except that I had needed emergency surgery with a transfusion in the Seychelles three months earlier. He scheduled me for more tests and two weeks later told me, "You have hepatitis C."

I thought he'd made a mistake. "But I feel fine," I said.

"Good," he replied. "We've caught your infection early, and I think we can keep you feeling fine."

Michael

The Silent Infection

This chapter explains how to get a diagnosis. Once you have been diagnosed, understanding your laboratory tests and what they mean to your health is very important. This chapter describes and explains these tests, what they mean, and what normal values are.

As you read in Chapter 1, hepatitis C is called a "silent" infection because affected people often do not feel sick. Because hepatitis C has few symptoms, many people have it for long periods before they are diagnosed, and this lag in diagnosis makes getting effective treatment more difficult. People with hepatitis C often feel minor symptoms such as some fatigue and vague discomfort in the right upper abdomen, but this can be ascribed to many other factors such as middle age, weight gain, emotional problems, and a host of other familiar ailments. We also saw in Chapter 1 that when first infected, some people have a brief fever and a few muscle aches. These are often ignored or discounted as a cold, flu, or another minor ailment.

Otherwise, most people with hepatitis C feel fine even as the virus and their antibodies are attacking their liver. Classic symptoms of hepatitis such as yellowed eyes and skin, severe itching, swelling of the legs and abdomen, nausea, and vomiting appear only later, when extensive liver damage has already taken place. This dearth of symptoms makes it difficult to get a timely diagnosis.

Most people who learn they have hepatitis C are diagnosed by accident. When they try to give blood, the screening tests that protect the blood supply from HCV contamination come back positive, and a letter from the blood bank informs them that they are infected with HCV. Regular medical examinations such as annual physicals often will not reveal hepatitis C, because the changes in your body tend to be subtle and gradual, even as your liver is being damaged. But blood tests for another medical problem sometimes reveal slightly elevated liver enzymes that lead an alert doctor to suspect that the person has hepatitis C.

EARLY WARNING. As you read in Chapter 1, an early diagnosis is preferable. As with many illnesses, from high blood pressure to cancer, the earlier you are diagnosed, the sooner and more effective treatment is likely to be. As you will read in Chapter 4, many scientists think that early treatment with the drug interferon works better than waiting until liver damage sets in. But if you don't know you are infected, you cannot take advantage of early treatment. Diet, supplements, herbs, and lifestyle changes also aid your body in fighting hepatitis C. But you cannot take specific steps to bolster your immune system and other natural defenses against hepatitis C if you do not know you are infected.

Finally, there are medications and other chemicals that people with liver problems should avoid. If you haven't been diagnosed, you may not realize that your smoking habit, your afternoon cocktail, or your job at the dry cleaner's may be hastening your liver damage.

Taking the Diagnostic Tests

WHO NEEDS AN HCV TEST?   First, decide whether you are at risk. If you think you may be, call your doctor for a blood test. As we saw in the last chapter, people who fall in the categories below are at increased risk:

- Anyone who had a blood transfusion or organ transplant before 1992 (or who had such a procedure in Canada before 1998)
- Anyone who is on dialysis
- Hemophiliacs who received clotting factor that was produced before 1987
- Anyone who has had a tattoo or piercing with tools that are not scrupulously cleaned
- Anyone who has used injected drugs or who has snorted cocaine
- Anyone who has had invasive medical procedures abroad or who hails from a country where HCV is common
- Anyone who has had multiple sexual partners *may* be at elevated risk
- The spouses or long-term partners of HCV-infected people should also be tested, although their lifetime risk is thought to be very low (1 to 5 percent)

There are probably other, unknown, risk factors. You may remember from Chapter 2 that no risk factors could be identified for 40 percent of the people who are diagnosed with hepatitis C.

If you have any of the foregoing risk factors, call your doctor for an HCV test. You may gain the peace of mind that comes from a negative test result. You may find that you were infected and are one of the minority who successfully quelled the infection. Or you may have an active infection and learn this early, so that your chances of avoiding serious liver damage are improved.

Diagnostic Tests

There are two types of blood tests for hepatitis C. The older, more common variety tests for and measures the presence of the virus-fighting antibodies you read about in Chapter 1. If antibodies to HCV are found, you are almost certainly infected with the virus. But newer tests search for the RNA virus itself. These tests measure the amount of the virus in your body as well. As you will read on page 64, there are six genotypes, or variants, of HCV; the viral tests can tell you what genotype you have.

All the modern HCV tests are very accurate, but they are not infallible. Each test yields a small number of false positives, which means a person is told she has hepatitis C when she does not. Tests can also generate false negatives, which means that a person who has hepatitis C is told that he does not carry the virus.

ELISA

Since 1989, *ELISA tests* have detected the presence of antibodies to HCV in the blood of infected people. The first ELISA test yielded many false positives and false negatives, but since 1996, refinements have made it very accurate. If you had an ELISA test before 1992, you should ask your doctor about whether taking today's more accurate test makes sense for you. Still, a few false positives slip though the new ELISA, mostly because about three of every one hundred people generate an enzyme called *superoxide dismutase* that can trigger a false-positive reaction from today's ELISA test. So your doctor may suggest confirming your positive test with a RIBA assay, described below.

RIBA Assays

RIBA assays indicate exactly which HCV antibodies are present. If your positive test is triggered by superoxide dismutase, RIBA will indicate this and you will know that you are not infected with hepatitis C. If RIBA indicates the presence of only one HCV antibody, you may or may not be infected, but if it reacts against two antibodies, you definitely are infected with HCV. In February 1999, the FDA approved a refinement to the RIBA assays. The RIBA HCV 3.0 Strip Immunoblot Assay (SIA) is better at eliminating the occasional false-positive results generated by the older test.

But neither ELISA nor RIBA directly measures the presence or the amount of the virus. This is important, because the 15 percent of people who clear the virus from their bodies without treatment may still have antibodies to HCV (and so may still have positive ELISA and RIBA tests), even though they are no longer infected.

RNA Assays

Directly testing for the presence of virus with *RNA assays* will resolve this ambiguous result. The RNA assay is also called an HCV-RNA test. RNA tests also tell you your *viral load*—how much virus is in your bloodstream. Viral load tends to be higher with people who have been infected for longer periods. It is also higher in people who were infected via intravenous blood exposure—blood-product transfusions or IV drug use. Intravenous blood exposure is how most Americans acquired HCV. Interferon treatment is less likely to work for people with high viral loads, so it is important for your doctor to know your viral load. Your laboratory report may give your viral load in viral particles per milliliter, for example, 2 million/ml. If it uses another, more confusing mathematical expression, ask your doctor to translate it for you.

TAKE-HOME TEST

In the summer of 1999, the FDA approved an over-the-counter test for hepatitis C, the **Hepatitis C Check,** that can be bought without a prescription and taken at home.

Here's how it works: You use an enclosed lancet to draw a drop of blood from your finger. You place the blood on the filter paper provided, then mail it to a laboratory for analysis. Your blood sample is assigned an identification number to preserve your confidentiality.

The laboratory uses the same FDA-licensed tests for antibodies to HCV that your doctor or local hospital uses. Four to ten business days later, you call a phone number to obtain the results from an automated phone system. If you request it, you can hear the results from a counselor. If you request it, you will be referred to a physician in your area for further counseling and treatment.

A study of 1,200 people who took the home kit found that its results were as accurate as those provided by laboratories and physicians. The Hepatitis C Check also protects your confidentiality, because your name need not be associated with the test. However, the home test for HCV is not as good as a diagnosis from your doctor for several reasons:

- Delivering shocking medical news via an automated telephone system is an ill-considered act that seems to discount the psychological trauma to which it subjects HCV-positive people. Infected people who do not understand that HCV is not a death sentence will suffer needless anguish.
- A person whose Hepatitis C Check is positive will still have to take a conventional HCV test and see a doctor for confirmatory tests. Home Access, the maker of Hepatitis C Check, says its automated messages and counselors warn people that they must follow up with a doctor. But this means that the test costs patients extra money instead of saving money.
- You can't know what the Hepatitis C Check diagnosis really

means. It reveals whether a person has ever contracted the hepatitis C virus. But is does not show whether it is active, acute, or chronic. If you are one of the 15 percent who clear the infection from their body without treatment, you will not learn this from the test results. Also, if you have been exposed within the past six months, the infection may not be revealed on the test.

Genotype

If you are HCV-infected, your doctor should send a blood sample to a laboratory for genotype testing to find out which of the six HCV genotypes you have. Knowing your genotype is helpful because genotype often affects your response to interferon treatment. Hepatitis C is classified into genotypes 1a, 1b, 2a, 2b, 3a, 3b, 4a, 4b, 5a, 5b, 6a, and 6b.

The prevalence of genotypes varies in different regions of the globe. Seventy-five percent of Americans have type 1a and 1b; the rest have types 2 or 3. Type 4 is prevalent in the Middle East and in eastern and central Africa; type 5 is found in regions of Canada and in southern Africa; and type 6 is prevalent in Asia. Unless you were born in or had invasive (blood-related) medical care outside North America, you probably need worry only about types 1 through 3.

As we will see in the next chapter, genotype 1 does not respond as well to interferon therapy as do the relatively rare types 2 and 3. In November 1997, the journal *Clinical Therapy* reported that 66.7 percent of the patients with genotype 2a had a good long-term response to interferon therapy, but only 7.1 percent of patients with genotype 1b infection did. But don't assume that interferon will not work for you if you are type 1: Some people of every genotype respond well to interferon, and if you have a low viral load, this increases the chances that interferon will help or cure you.

Other genetic factors, such as *quasispecies,* also come into play. Because hepatitis C mutates so rapidly, copies of the virus that differ from each other are soon circulating in the blood. These are called quasispecies, meaning that the infection is caused by several distinct but related genetic strains of the virus. The longer you have had HCV, the greater the number of quasi- species that have evolved in your body. People with the greatest number of quasispecies have the poorest response to interferon therapy. People with the most quasispecies also have worse liver disease. But some experts are unconvinced that quasispecies *cause* the poorer outcomes, and point out that no causal relation- ship has yet been proven.

Doctors do not send your blood to a laboratory to measure the number of quasispecies your body harbors. This is partly because no quasipecies-based treatment modifications are yet known to improve the outcome. Hopefully, the role of quasispecies will be clarified in the next three to five years, and treatment based on this additional information will help more people with hepati- tis C respond to treatment.

Don't forget that despite the prevalence of a "poor" genotype and increasing numbers of quasispecies as time goes on, most people with hepatitis C will never develop life-threatening liver disease.

Co-Infection

You may have more than one type of hepatitis. In July 1999, the *New England Journal of Medicine* reported that the Policlinico Universitario in Messina, Italy, found that 66 of their 200 hepa- titis C patients also harbored the hepatitis B virus. The *Journal* determined that a "hidden," that is, hard-to-diagnose, type of hepa- titis B virus frequently infects people who have chronic hepati- tis C liver disease. So if you have hepatitis C, you should get a *DNA-PCR test* for hepatitis B as well.

Some people are co-infected with HIV and HCV; in fact, peo- ple with HIV are at higher risk for hepatitis C because their im- mune systems are weakened. Co-infected people are in especial danger because their immune-system damage allows HCV to spread quickly and escalates the rate of liver damage, advanced cirrhosis, cancer, and the need for liver transplants. But a person can increase her chances of escaping such serious liver injury and decrease her risks of dying from hepatitis C by having an HIV test, then seeing her doctor regularly for monitoring tests.

I Have Hepatitis C. Now What?

Once you have been diagnosed with hepatitis C, you will begin a lifelong regimen of important tests. They will tell you and your doctor how your liver is faring with the infection: Is your liver clearing the virus from your body? Are you developing fibrosis?

Looking at Your Liver

The tests just described are essential for an early diagnosis, but they can also be deceptive because they do not portray a complete picture of your liver disease. A person whose liver is still functioning vigorously and who remains pretty healthy may have a high amount of HCV and genotype 1. So can someone on the brink of cirrhosis. To get a direct assessment of how hepatitis C is affecting *your* health, you doctor will want to take a look, or more likely several looks, at your liver. He or she uses various technologies to do so.

IMAGING SCANS. Ultrasound and CT scans are common, safe ways for your doctor to see your liver. Doctors often start with ultrasound, which is the same technique doctors use to peer at developing fetuses. Sound waves beyond our hearing range penetrate and bounce off liver tissues. The ultrasound machine records and translates these sounds into live visual images of the liver. Your physician can see the liver's size, any changes in its architecture or tissue density, and any areas of fibrosis or cirrhosis. He or she can also see the condition of the liver's ducts and blood vessels.

The next step is often a CT, or *computerized tomography,* scan. These are also called CAT, or *computerized axial tomogra-*

phy, scans. Computerized tomography uses low-level radiation to form a static image that is akin to a very sophisticated X-ray. CT scans give an image of any plane inside the person's body—a cross-sectional slice. These offer more information than ultrasound, because the image is sharply defined and is not distorted by fluid or air. This clearer view yields a more consistently accurate assessment of liver problems such as cirrhosis or tumors than ultrasound images.

BIOPSY. Unlike the scans, a liver biopsy is *invasive*—the doctor goes inside your body. He or she removes a small sample of your liver tissue for analysis. You will be asked to sign a consent form because the biopsy is technically a surgical procedure. But it is a simple, quick, outpatient procedure performed with a local anesthetic and an additional painkiller, if needed. Your liver has no sensory nerves and cannot feel pain, but the surrounding tissues can.

The doctor inserts a needle directly into your liver, then uses it to take a small sample of tissue. He or she sends it to a pathologist, who looks at it with his naked eye and records its appearance. He then places cells from the sample under the microscope to confirm that you have hepatitis and not another infection or condition that mimics it; this is called the *histologic examination*. If there are areas of fibrosis or cirrhosis, the pathologist reports them so you and your doctor can locate them and devise a treatment strategy.

The doctor will want you to remain for a few hours of observation because a relatively few people experience complications such as prolonged bleeding from the biopsy site. Serious complications are rare, but one person in a thousand dies from the procedure, so a biopsy is not risk-free.

The very word *biopsy* is frightening because of its associations with cancer. Remember that unlike a biopsy that is looking for cancer, the biopsies you will undergo are to track the progression of a disease that you already know you have. The first, or "baseline," biopsy allows the doctor to evaluate the presence or extent of liver damage so he or she will know how best to treat you. You will undergo subsequent biopsies to look for evidence of changes in the liver. These are rarely due to cancer. As you read in Chapter 1, the natural progression of the disease is to fibrosis and cirrhosis, so the biopsy is taken to judge whether liver disease is progressing, and specifically to look for evidence of cirrhosis.

You will see your doctor at least once every six months. But how often your doctor checks for signs of cirrhosis will vary according to your risk factors; the disease progresses at a different rate for everyone.

Understanding Your Laboratory Reports

Your liver-function tests are called by confusing acronyms that stand for unpronounceable chemicals. Their values are written in cryptic medical shorthand. In short, they sound intimidating. Yet, in order to take an active role in your own care, you should learn what your test results mean, and this chapter will help you to do just that.

This chapter will explain the purpose of each test and the basic information hidden in your laboratory-test numbers. There are lots of technical terms and so many acronyms that a hepatitis C laboratory profile looks like a sheet full of Scrabble tiles. But a little patience pays off in understanding what the laboratory tests are saying about your liver's condition. You do not have to know all the names and you certainly can't expect to memorize the normal test values given in the tables on the following pages. So don't try to remember all the details. Instead, just remember that the information is here, in plain English. You can always turn to this chapter for reference when you get new test results. After a while, the more common tests will become familiar to you and you will understand whether your results are good without having to look them up.

Your doctor should go over every report with you. If he or she doesn't offer to, ask. You should also keep your own personal medical chart. You can do this simply by using a loose-leaf note-book where you can store copies of your lab reports and pre-scriptions. Always ask your doctor for a copy of your laboratory tests for your notebook. Write down any new symptoms and any questions you have for your doctor. This will help you to see pat-terns in your symptoms, which will help you and your caregivers to decide what is working and is not working for you.

Once diagnosed, you will probably be referred to a gastro-enterologist or a hepatologist (liver specialist) who has a lot of experience in treating people with hepatitis C. If he is not an ex-perienced specialist, I suggest you turn to the beginning of Chapter 4, because its first section tells you how to find an expe-rienced doctor.

One of the first notations you will see is called *liver staging.* Hepatologists place patients with hepatitis C into categories, or *stages,* based upon the degree of fibrosis, or scarring revealed by the scans and biopsy.

- **Stage 0** means you have no noticeable inflammation or fi-brosis; you have a normal-looking liver.
- Early, or **stage I,** disease is characterized by liver inflamma-tion only.
- Intermediate, or **stage II,** disease entails some localized fibrosis.
- Livers with **stage III** disease have moderate fibrosis to se-vere fibrosis connected by "bridges" of scarred liver tissue.
- **Stage IV** is *cirrhosis,* or extensive fibrosis that distorts the shape and impedes the function of the liver. Most stage IV patients eventually need a liver transplant.

Monitoring Tests

These measure important proteins and enzymes to determine how well your liver is standing up to the onslaught of the virus. These blood tests measure bilirubin, albumin, clotting factors, and the quantities of various blood cells. As you read in Chap-ter 1, the liver manufactures these substances; a blood test that measures them also gives an indirect measure of liver damage. The discussion of laboratory test values below indicates a range of normal test values. But there is much variation in the meaning of laboratory tests, so it is important to discuss your results with your doctor. Only then can you understand their meaning for you.

	NORMAL	MODERATE	SEVERE
Bilirubin	0.3–1.2 mg/dl	1.2–2.5 mg/dl	greater than 2.5 mg/dl
Albumin	5.0 g/liter	5.0–3.5 g/liter	less than 3.5 mg/dl
Prothrombin time	less than 14 seconds		17+ seconds
Ammonia	less than 50 mcg/dl		

Enzyme Levels

As the liver suffers injury, the blood levels of various enzymes rise. In Chapter 1, I likened the liver to a factory complex. Enzymes are *protein catalysts* that help your liver's biochemical reactions to proceed quickly. They are supposed to remain within the liver, but as your liver suffers increasing injury, they leach out into the surrounding bloodstream. Among the enzymes you will be periodically tested for are:

ALANINE AMINOTRANSFERASE, OR ALT, LEVELS (these used to be called SGPT tests and some reports still use this term, too). Rising ALT levels show a *continuing increase* in liver cell destruction, but interpreting these is tricky. Your ALT levels rise from the time you are infected until cirrhosis appears. But the rise is so gradual that the ALT levels of most people with cirrhosis remain within normal limits. What is important is the relative increase, not the absolute level.

	NORMAL	MODERATE	SEVERE
Men	0–31 units/liter	31–200 units/liter	200+ units/liter
Women	9–24 units/liter	24–200 units/liter	200+ units/liter

Your ALT levels may stop rising for a time when cirrhosis develops, because when liver cells die and are replaced by the scar tissue of cirrhosis, those cells stop releasing enzymes. The bottom line: Rising ALT levels always indicate liver cell destruction; static or falling ALT levels often but do not always mean improvement. Many medications, including barbiturates, chlorpromazine, codeine, griseofulvin, isoniazid, meperidine, methyldopa, morphine, narcotic analgesics, nitrofurantoin, para-aminosalicylic acid, phenothiazines, phenytoin, tetracycline, aspirin and other salicylates can raise ALT levels, too.

ASPARTATE AMINOTRANSFERASE, OR AST LEVELS (these used to be called SGOT tests and some reports still use this term, too). AST levels also rise as hepatitis injures your liver.

NORMAL	MODERATE	SEVERE
10–37 units/liter	38–200 units/liter	200+ units/liter

GAMMA-GLUTAMYL TRANSFERASE, OR GGT LEVELS. There is usually no increase in GGT levels until cirrhosis develops. Then you *may* see a modest increase from normal values.

NORMAL	MODERATE	SEVERE
7–59 units/liter	60–200 units/liter	200+ units/liter

ALKALINE PHOSPHATASE LEVELS. There is usually no increase in alkaline phosphatase levels until cirrhosis develops.

Then you may see a modest increase from normal values. If you are taking barbiturates, chlorpropamide, halothane, isoniazid, methyldopa, oral contraceptives, phenothiazines or phenytoin, these can inflate alkaline phosphatase levels. Rising GGT and alkaline phosphatase levels can also reflect liver problems other than hepatitis C.

	NORMAL	MODERATE	SEVERE
Men	90–117 units/liter	117–200 units/liter	200–239+ units/liter
Women under 45	100–117 units/liter	117–196 units/liter	196+ units/liter
Women over 45	87–150 units/liter	150–200 units/liter	200–250 units/liter

WBC, HCT, and Platelets

The acronym **WBC** refers to your *white blood cell count,* the number of infection-fighting white blood cells in a standard sample of blood. The WBC can indicate moderate cirrhosis, portal hypertension, or another complication of hepatitis C. So can a low HCT. HCT stands for *hematocrit,* which is the percentage of blood made up of red blood cells. Platelets are cell fragments that play an important role in blood clotting.

	NORMAL	MODERATE	SEVERE
WBC	6,000+	3,000–6,000	fewer than 3,000
Hematocrit	40+	35–39	fewer than 35
Platelets	150,000+	100,000–150,000	fewer than 100,000

Blood Protein Tests

Enzyme levels indicate the presence of liver damage, but to find out details of how your liver is working, you need to look at the quality and quantity of blood proteins and the other substances your liver makes. Blood protein tests tell you how extensively the liver's ability to produce, store, and distribute these substances has been compromised.

ALBUMIN. The liver synthesizes albumin, a special protein that maintains the body's precise fluid balance. Although other diseases can lower albumin levels, very low levels can mean your liver disease has been escalating for at least a month. When albumin levels fall below 25 grams per liter, plasma diffuses from the veins and arteries into tissues. This causes swelling in the legs (edema) and in the abdomen (ascites). Ascites is a serious complication.

PROTHROMBIN AND OTHER CLOTTING FACTORS. The liver must constantly generate prothrombin, which helps the blood coagulate and clot. When the liver loses the ability to make these clotting factors, levels drop quickly—within twenty-four to forty-eight hours. A blood test will show this drop. People with low prothrombin levels bruise and bleed easily, like hemophiliacs. Like hemophiliacs, they may need to take clotting factors, which were described in the last chapter. The *prothrombin time (PT) test* indicates how long it takes blood to clot. This tells your doctor how efficiently your clotting factors are working. As you can see from the table on page 70, a longer-than-normal prothrombin time means that your blood's ability to clot has fallen. If your prothrombin climbs high enough, you risk symptoms such as blood blisters, bleeding gums, and dangerous internal hemorrhaging. Sometimes a vitamin K injection will allow your liver to start making clotting factor again. If your liver doesn't respond, you may need a liver transplant.

BILIRUBIN. This is a yellowish pigment that leaches out of dying red blood cells. The healthy liver excretes bilirubin into bile. In people with hepatitis C, bilirubin levels typically go up and down. But a bilirubin level that soars and remains high can mean trouble for someone with hepatitis C. This means that many more red blood cells are dying than are being replaced, or it means that the liver is too badly injured to do its job of recycling the bilirubin into bile. Anti-malarial drugs, ascorbic acid (vitamin C), epinephrine, histidine, isoproterenol, levodopa, methyldopa, rifampin, streptomycin, sulfa drugs, theophylline, and tyrosine can skew bilirubin test results.

Unfortunately, once bilirubin remains elevated to 3 milligrams per deciliter or higher, light-skinned people no longer need a blood test to tell them that something is wrong. The excess bilirubin turns the skin and whites of the eyes yellow, a condition called *jaundice*. Dark-skinned people, including African Americans, also suffer this skin color change, but at the early stages of jaundice, the changes may be too subtle for anyone but a liver expert to notice. Dark-skinned people can notice jaundice in the palms and soles before detecting it in rest of their skin. At the same time that the skin turns yellowish, your stools begin to look pale or whitish. This is because the bilirubin is lingering in your blood and tissues, instead of being excreted into the stools. So they lose their characteristic dark brown color.

Complete Blood Count

This test can indicate the degree of scarring in your liver and the presence of portal hypertension, which was discussed in Chapter 1. The backup of blood flow in your spleen creates pressure, just as the water backup forces the walls of the garden hose to balloon out. This pressure makes the spleen balloon. The blood cells are trapped in the ballooning spleen, and because the cells cannot enter the blood vessels, the blood cell counts fall quite low.

Hormones

Your doctor will probably test your thyroid function when you are diagnosed and again when you begin interferon treatment. People with hepatitis C often suffer from underlying thyroid disease, because the liver is an important generator of hormones and the thyroid is an important hormonal organ. As explained in Chapter 4, interferon therapy can cause or exacerbate a thyroid condition.

If your cirrhosis progresses to stage III or stage IV, you will be vulnerable to other hormonal imbalances. The sex hormones that govern menstruation, sperm production, and gonadal health can be affected. People with severe cirrhosis acquire abnormal secondary sex characteristics such as *gynecomastia,* breast development in men.

Interpreting the Scores

There is not always a one-to-one correspondence between a single score and the condition of your liver. For example, a person with mild inflammation and a person with limited cirrhosis can share the same ALT score. It's the pattern of your scores over time and the combined portrait of your liver presented by all the tests and a biopsy that tell you and your doctor how your liver is faring and how it is responding to treatment.

I am a critical care nurse. In October of 1998, we had a blood drive at the hospital and I decided to donate. It had been at least nine or ten years since I gave blood. Two months later I got a lovely letter from the blood bank telling me I had hepatitis C. I was devastated. Immediately I went to my family doctor and had blood work done. I know several hep. C nurses and through them I found a good gastroenterologist and had more blood work done then.

My "labs" are perfect . . . all within normal limits. I have no elevation of my liver enzymes. But my liver biopsy shows bridging necrosis, and I have moderate portal hypertension.

My genotype is 2a and my viral load is not too high.

How this came to be is a total mystery to me. But I'm not dwelling on that; I'm focusing on learning about all these tests and making sure I do everything I can to get well. Now in about three weeks I'll go on interferon and ribavirin. Scary stuff, those side effects, but if I get rid of the virus, it will be worth it.

Georgia

Now that you understand what hepatitis C is, how to minimize the risk of contracting it and spreading it, and how laboratory tests illuminate how the virus has affected you, you are ready to learn about treatment. Like Georgia, you need to make a decision about interferon therapy, the chief conventional medication used against hepatitis C. The next chapter will explain everything you need to know.

For more information

Online Sources

Hepatitis C Fact Sheet
www.cdc.gov/ncidod/diseases/hepatitis/c/fact.htm
A fact sheet published by the Centers for Disease Control; it is also available by calling (404) 332-4555.

Hepatitis Education Project
www.halcyon.com/jevo/Hep
Publishes a quarterly newsletter and educational materials.

Evaluating Blood Test Results, Liver Biopsies, and Other Diagnostic Tests: Normal Value Ranges for Blood Tests
http://www.askemilyss.com/Livrtest.htm

Hepatitis C—Blood and Other Tests
http://village.vossnet.co.uk/c/crina/pag-tests-menu.html

"Common Laboratory Tests in Liver Diseases," by Howard J. Worman, M.D.
http://cpmcnet.columbia.edu/dept/gi/labtests.html

Hepatitis Central's Viral Load Chart
Click on "What is Viral Load," http://hepatitiscentral.com/hcv/hepatitis/loadchart.html
This site interprets the different manners in which your viral load may be reported.

CBC Blood Chemistry Definitions
www.carbon.com/cbcblood.htm

Dr. Greenson's Gastrointestinal and Liver Pathology Extravaganza
www.path.med.umich.edu/users/greenson/M2liverlecture.html

This is a lecture given by a pathologist to medical students, complete with slides.

The Effects of Drugs on Laboratory Values

www.li.net/~edhayes/labtestmain2.html

This is a list of drugs that can distort your liver test results.

CHAPTER FOUR

Conventional Treatment:
Cure for a Fortunate Few

*The wise man in the storm prays to God, not for safety
from danger, but for deliverance from fear.*
—*Ralph Waldo Emerson,* Journals

Congratulations on having gotten this far. You now understand
that hepatitis C is a serious disease that you will almost certainly
have to live with, not die from. You understand the importance of
an early diagnosis, of genotypes, how you can acquire the virus,
and how to protect others. You understand what the different
laboratory tests mean and know that you can refer back to Chapter 3, which offers detailed information to help you put your lab
values in context.

Most important, you understand that this book can give you a
clear factual background and explain treatment options for
HCV, but that it is critically important to discuss treatment decisions with your personal physician. He or she is the only expert
who can advise what is right *for you.*

Overview

Scarcely a decade has passed since hepatitis C was identified,
so it is disappointing but not surprising that there is no cure or

vaccine for HCV. Unfortunately, most people with HCV will find that there is not even a medical treatment that works well for them—yet.

The linchpin of conventional therapy is *interferon,* either alone or in combination with other drugs. However, interferon leaves a lot to be desired. It permanently arrests hepatitis in only 15 percent of people with HCV, costs roughly five thousand dollars for six months of treatment that will probably have to be repeated, and its side effects are profound, although manageable. But there are promising new treatment trends, including longer therapy with higher interferon doses and a slew of other drugs that are undergoing clinical and laboratory tests.

Whether and when to take interferon is a complex decision. You and your doctor must consider the level of virus in your blood, your genotype, the condition of your liver, and your iron levels. Deciding which variation on the theme of interferon treatment you should choose can also be complicated. Because many scientific studies lump together hepatitis C patients of differing genotypes, stages of liver damage, and virus concentrations, comparing results can be like comparing apples and oranges.

First, Choose a Doctor

You are about to venture into a sea of complex information and interacting risks. To sail the right course, you need the guidance of a physician who knows you, your medical history, your state of health, and your state of mind. Your doctor will help you to accurately weigh the risks and benefits of any particular treatment *for you*.

Your physician also plays an important role as your primary medical advocate. He or she is invaluable in treating side effects, making referrals to other professionals, coordinating your medications, and helping you make decisions. She can ease your entrée into appropriate treatment, whether it involves psychological support, alternative approaches, cutting-edge therapy, or a clinical trial. In the unlikely event that you should need a transplant, having a savvy, well-connected physician can be a matter of life and death.

> I am a veteran and had been going through the usual VA routine and wasn't getting very far. No medication at all, and they told me little. They didn't even mention interferon until I brought it up.
>
> What I did was to spend a lot of time online after I got the diagnosis, trying to learn about the disease. I then found a doctor on a Web site at Vanderbilt who was doing research. So I e-mailed him and he invited me in to see him. This doctor saw me and took me on as a patient after he found I had studied the disease and was intent on getting well. He pushed the envelope a little and got me on combo treatment. That is not easy through the VA because the drugs are so expensive. I think he got me on as part of a test. I've been seeing him since.
>
> Tyrone

Choose Your Physician Carefully

You would do well to adopt Tyrone's strategy: Educate yourself and find a good physician-partner. Because conventional medicine cannot offer most people with hepatitis C effective treatment, many people are tempted to research and coordinate their medical care on their own. Don't. Navigating the jungle of hard-to interpret medical information is like trying to travel solo in a war-torn foreign land without knowing the language. You can do it, but not very well and not very safely. So invest some time in choosing the best doctor you can find.

SPECIALTY.   Your doctor must be an expert on hepatitis C. This usually means he or she is a board-certified gastroenterologist, who specializes in disorders of the digestive system, or a hepatologist, a doctor who specializes in liver disease.

EXPERIENCE.   Your doctor must also be experienced in treating people with HCV. Ask how many he or she has treated. There is no magic number, but look for a doctor who says the majority of his or her patients have hepatitis.

UNIVERSITY AFFILIATION. Having a physician with experience in treating hepatitis C is more important, but doctors with a university affiliation sometimes find it easier to keep up with current research and resources, such as clinical trials of new drugs.

ALTERNATIVE-FRIENDLY. If you think you may want to pursue alternative treatment, be sure to choose a physician who is receptive to, or better yet, has expertise in, such treatment.

NAMING NAMES. You should ask your primary physician or internist to suggest the names of specialists. Hepatitis C support-group members are another excellent source of good physicians' names. The American Liver Foundation will give you the name of experts in your area, but won't evaluate them for you. You can also call medical-center referral lines in the Yellow Pages, but they recommend only their own physicians.

INTERVIEW YOUR PROSPECTIVE DOCTOR. You should "interview" a few prospective doctors before choosing one. You may have to have to pay for these office visits, but think of it as an investment in your good health.

Ask the questions below, as well as any others that are important to you:

- How long have you been treating people with HCV? How many such patients have you treated?
- How do you feel about treating a patient who wants to be an active participant in planning his or her own treatment?
- How often do you refer people to clinical trials of new drugs?
- What can you offer me if interferon doesn't work for me?
- How do you feel about alternative therapy? Do you make referrals to alternative practitioners?

- (If you are older than 60) How would my age affect the treatment you recommend? Would it preclude a prescription for interferon?

You will probably need emotional support, because depression, sleep disorders, and fatigue are sometimes caused or worsened by interferon therapy. So don't discount the emotional factor. During your conversation, you should sense genuine concern and acceptance. This rapport can't always be quantified; you will have to pay attention to your "gut feelings."

Finally, don't forget the practical details:

- Make sure your ideal doctor accepts your insurance plan.
- Is the office too far away? You may be very fatigued or even unable to drive at some point in your treatment.
- What are the staff members like? Brusque, insensitive, disorganized staff can make the most empathetic healer's office a nightmare.
- Is the doctor so good that he or she is just *too* busy? Find out what the average wait is for an appointment.

What Is Interferon?

Now that you have a doctor, you and your doctor can decide together whether you should try interferon. But first, you need to understand what interferon is.

We've known about interferon since 1957. Scientists observed that when our bodies are infected with a virus, the infected cells produce special proteins, collectively called interferon, that protect other cells from infection. This substance gets its name from the fact that it directly *interferes* with viral replication as well as indirectly interferes by stimulating the immune system to fight infections.

When researchers discovered that liver damage compromises that organ's ability to produce enough interferon, they hypothesized that administering interferon might help the liver to heal itself. Their hypothesis proved correct.

Interferon prevents the HCV virus from making more copies of itself. This can slow or prevent liver deterioration. This also causes liver alanine transaminase, or ALT, levels to fall. ALT is an enzyme that is released into the blood when liver cells are injured, so higher-than-normal levels indicate ongoing liver damage. ALT levels are used in concert with other tests to measure interferon's efficacy: When they fall to normal levels, doctors surmise that liver damage may have ceased. But interferon cannot undo liver damage that has already taken place, so it is most effective when taken in the early course of liver disease, before fibrosis or cirrhosis has set in. Interferon's usefulness is not just measured by whether you attain a "cure": Interferon reduces inflammation and retards liver damage, buying you time in which a better treatment will certainly emerge.

There are three major groups of interferons—alpha, beta, and gamma. Alpha interferons combat viral infections most efficiently, beta is less efficient, and gamma interferon doesn't help people with HCV at all. Alpha interferons are further subdivided into:

- Roferon—alpha 2a interferon
- Intron A—alpha 2b interferon, which can be used for up to two years
- Wellferon—alpha n1 interferon
- Alferon-N—alpha n3 interferon
- Rebetron—a new combination of interferon and ribavirin

The Selective Bullet

Interferon stops liver damage in half of the people who take it. These people are called "responders." If interferon can help you, you will respond within the first eight weeks of treatment. This is why your doctor will recommend that you discontinue treatment if your liver enzymes have not fallen by the third or fourth month of treatment.

Those who initially respond have cleared only the first hurdle. Nearly everyone will relapse a few months after they stop taking interferon. Their enzymes will rise again and so will the levels of virus in their blood. When they are re-treated, probably with the more powerful Rebetron therapy, their enzymes will almost certainly fall again. But relapse is so common after that, that treatment may be nearly continuous for those who can tolerate the side effects. In the end, interferon can slow liver damage, but it gives only 15 percent of patients the dramatic, *sustained* drop to normal enzyme levels and undetectable viral load that can mean permanent victory over HCV.

Should You Try Interferon?

Are the uncertain benefits of interferon worth the certain physical, emotional, and financial costs? Yes, usually they are. But this is one of those maddening cases where there is no blanket medical answer. You and your doctor will make that decision after weighing your liver disease status, your current state of health, your risk factors, and your own feelings.

Early interferon treatment is definitely recommended for people who have high levels of the virus. These tend to be people who acquired HCV via transfusion, hemophilia treatment, or drug use. Their liver damage is likely to progress relatively quickly and they cannot afford to await.

DO YOU NEED INTERFERON NOW? Interferon's expense is partnered with side effects that are probably worse than your current symptoms. These drawbacks make it tempting to wait for something more efficient to come along.

One factor you must weigh is the risk that your hepatitis will progress to cirrhosis or liver cancer. Of every one hundred people diagnosed with HCV, as few as twenty develop cirrhosis. As few as five will develop liver cancer. Most people with HCV will never develop either. For most people, HCV progresses slowly, so your doctor may recommend "watchful waiting." If so, she will examine and test you regularly, and you and she will consider treatment if and when your liver show signs of deterioration. As one physician summarized, "If I had a biopsy that showed no fibrosis, I'd rather wait five years until a better drug comes along with far fewer side effects."

Yet waiting carries costs, too. There is evidence that people who begin interferon therapy early have a better chance of responding well. And recent studies suggest that for some people, such as those co-infected with HIV, early, aggressive treatment is the key to preventing liver damage.

The above factors determine whether you *need* interferon. But there is also the question of whether interferon is likely to work for you, as indicated by your genotype, blood levels of the virus, and iron levels.

In order to be considered for interferon therapy, you must have:

- **Infection with HCV** as evinced by the HCV-RNA assay or an antibody test.
- **Signs of *chronic* hepatitis.** This means ALT levels that remain at least one and a half times as great as normal levels for at least six months. But as you'll see on page 92, people with *acute* hepatitis are increasingly being found eligible.
- **Good overall health.** Another serious chronic medical condition such as diabetes or cancer usually precludes you from interferon treatment until the condition has been cured or controlled. Some essential medications for other chronic conditions interact dangerously with interferon. But people who are infected with HIV can take interferon, particularly during the early stages when they remain in good health.

A liver biopsy should show a liver with signs of chronic hepatitis but with no cirrhosis or fibrosis, because such seriously damaged livers may be unable to weather the stress to which interferon would subject it. If you have signs of liver failure, including bleeding varices or ascites, you are not eligible.

On the other end of the spectrum, if your biopsy shows few or no signs of liver damage, your doctor may feel that your liver is too mildly damaged to risk the side effects of interferon therapy. However, because recent research suggests that undamaged livers may have the best chance of sustained recovery with interferon, be sure you discuss this development with your doctor if he is reluctant to recommend interferon.

If you are a hemophiliac, are co-infected with HIV, or were infected by a transfusion or long-term drug use, liver damage may progress quickly, so you and your doctor may want to proceed with interferon even if you have few or no signs of liver damage.

How Interferon Is Used

If you and your doctor decide to try interferon, he or she will determine which type is most likely to work well for you, then tell you how often and for how long you will need to take it.

Interferon is injected, and most people must take it for six months to a year. Until recently, most people took three weekly doses, but the recommended dosing schedule changed to five times a week in mid-1999. You will probably take 5 million units—five thousandths of a gram five times a week, usually Monday through Friday. However, your doctor may start you on a lower or a higher dosing schedule.

You will have to learn to give yourself the injections. But even if you dislike needles—and who doesn't?—you may find the injections easier than you think. For one thing, you inject yourself just under the skin. This is very different from the painful probing for a "good" vein that often accompanies having blood taken. It's also less painful and difficult than the deep muscle shots given for flu vaccine.

When my doctor said I'd have to give myself injections, my palms began to sweat. I dreaded it. I'd always prayed that I wouldn't become diabetic like my father because I didn't see how I could ever give myself injections. When Dr. Lawrence pulled out a hypodermic needle, I was ready to bolt for the door. Until she rolled a scarred, bruised grapefruit over the desk toward me. I was shocked. "What's *that* for?" I blurted. The look on my face must have been funny, because she laughed.

"Practice!"

She showed me how it was done once or twice, pinching the skin of the fruit and inserting the needle at a right angle. Then she let me inject the grapefruit as she coached. The practice made me feel more confident, and I must say, I caught on quickly. When I injected myself, it wasn't so bad after all. She asked me to stay in the treatment room for a half hour just to make sure I felt all right afterward. Now I inject myself every weekday without a thought. It's easy.

Terry

Your doctor or a nurse should monitor your first dose in the very unlikely event that you have a reaction to the interferon. Your doctor will want to see you regularly to test your liver enzymes and the level of virus in your blood and to monitor any side effects.

Store interferon in the refrigerator; your medicine cabinet is too warm and moist. Make sure you understand how to rotate injection sites and to keep the drug sterile in order to avoid an infection, because if you develop an infection and need antibiotics, you may have to discontinue interferon. During interferon treatment, keep the lines of communication open between you and your doctor. A 1992 Harvard School of Public Health survey revealed that most patients leave their doctors' offices without understanding instructions for taking and storing their medications. Because hepatitis C, interferon, and even the anxiety of being ill can interfere with your ability to concentrate, make sure that you understand what you are supposed to do. Ask your doctor to put instructions in writing or for patient pamphlets that explain dosing and side effects. Buy a small notebook and use it to note questions and side effects.

Assessing Your Progress

Your doctor will order blood tests frequently while you are taking interferon. These will tell you whether interferon is helping you and how the level of liver enzymes is responding. Because interferon can hamper production of blood cells, particularly of the body's infection-fighting white cells (polymorphonuclear leuko-cytes) these tests will also ensure that interferon is not danger-ously weakening your immune function. The higher the interferon dose, the more dramatically blood cell production is depressed.

In general, you will see an improvement in ALT levels and in the amount of virus as measured by the HCV-RNA test. But the relationship between your test results and your liver health can be complex.

You will not always see a one-to-one correspondence between the change in enzyme levels and the change in liver function. A large drop in ALT levels may not mean a large increase in liver function. Conversely, a small ALT change may accompany a large improvement in liver health.

Blood tests will also reveal whether you are the one person in five who develops thyroid imbalance as a result of interferon therapy. The thyroid, a two-inch gland in your neck, secretes hor-mones that help regulate metabolism. An underactive, or *hypo-active,* thyroid causes lethargy; sluggishness; dry, brittle hair and nails; and weight gain. An overactive, or *hyperactive,* thyroid can cause weight loss, nervousness, sleeping difficulties, bulg-ing eyes, and diarrhea. These imbalances are rarely serious, but may become permanent over a long course of interferon. It is worth the risk: Unlike hepatitis C, thyroid problems are consis-tently treatable with artificial hormones.

IS INTERFERON WORKING FOR YOU?   To find out, your doctor looks at three main indicators during interferon therapy. These tests should be familiar to you from the last chapter:

- **ALT levels.** The most important determinant of success is whether the injury to your liver begins to abate. Falling ALT (alanine aminotransferase) levels tell you this. When ALT levels fall within the normal range, your liver disease has stopped progressing.
- **HCV-PCR tests.** The levels of hepatitis C virus in your blood should also begin to diminish if treatment is working.

PCR (polymerase chain reaction) assays will indicate this, so the test results are referred to as HCV-PCR tests.
- **Post-treatment biopsy.** After treatment ends, your doctor will biopsy your liver and examine it microscopically for lessening of inflammation and fibrosis. These are signs that your liver's health has improved.

Your Response Quotient

If interferon returns your ALT levels to normal within four months of beginning treatment, you are a *complete responder*. In four or five people who achieve normal ALT levels, the HCV level in their blood plummets, too, and the virus falls to "undetectable" levels by the end of therapy. This means that the medication kills off enough of the virus that conventional tests cannot detect it. The virus has not completely vanished, but it is now so sparse as to be relatively harmless. The problem is that it remains in the body and might begin to reproduce and proliferate again at any time.

For a lucky 15 percent of people on interferon, the level of HCV in the blood remains undetectable and the ALT levels remain normal after treatment is discontinued. These people have a *sustained response,* the best outcome. If a sustained response lasts for four or five years, you may be cured of hepatitis C.

But most complete responders will relapse again after interferon re-treatment stops. Relapsers need additional treatment for an additional six months to three years.

In some other people, ALT levels fall significantly, but not to normal levels. These people are called *partial responders*. Usually the ALT must fall as low as one and a half times the normal level for the person to be considered a partial responder. Their PCR-HCVs show that the HCV has not disappeared from their blood, and when interferon treatment is stopped, the ALT rises again, indicating that liver damage has resumed.

Half of the people who take interferon do not respond at all. The high ALT levels of these *nonresponders* persist, and the level of HCV in their blood does not diminish.

FOR WHOM DOES INTERFERON WORK BEST?   Unfortunately, data from clinical studies have not been precise enough to allow doctors to pinpoint those who will and will not benefit from interferon. But doctors have identified some "success" factors. People who benefit from interferon therapy share:

- **Relatively low levels of virus** in the blood. Among other things, this means that interferon works best for those who were more recently infected.
- Other **important laboratory values** should fall within these ranges: *albumin* (a protein produced by the liver and normally released into the blood) greater than 3.5 grams per deciliter; *bilirubin* (a component of bile) lower than 4 milligrams per deciliter; *hemoglobin* (the iron-rich oxygen-carrying component of blood) greater than 11 grams per deciliter; *platelet* (blood-cell particle that promotes healing) count greater than 70,000 per microliter; *prothrombin time* (the time needed for the blood to clot) more than 3 seconds longer than normal; *white blood cell count* greater than 3,300 per microliter.
- **A genotype other than 1.** Doctors do not decide who should have interferon strictly according to genotype, because some people of every genotype will respond. But about 60 percent of those with HCV genotype 2a and 2b respond, 40 percent of those with genotype 3 respond, and a little over 25 percent of the other genotypes respond, except for genotype 1: Fewer than 10 percent of people with genotype 1 respond.
- **Tolerance for long-term interferon treatment.** People willing and able to undergo treatment for longer periods at higher doses maximize their chances of a sustained response or even a cure, according to a 1997 meta-analysis. A meta-analysis is a painstaking analysis of a large number of clinical studies in an attempt to find new treatment-response relationships. This analysis found that taking interferon for at least a year yielded higher rates of sustained response. The doses taken by those in the studies were one and a half

times the usual dose taken a few years ago, but this is actually a little lower than most of today's recommended doses.

INTERFERON DOES NOT WORK WELL FOR:

- **People whose ALT levels are normal** although they have hepatitis C.
- **Pregnant women.** The effect of interferon on unborn children is unknown, so women of childbearing age should use a contraceptive until six months after completing treatment, and men who take interferon should use a condom.
- **Older people.** Many experts worry that older people are less likely to respond and may be less well able to tolerate interferon's side effects. But all sixty-five-year-olds are not alike, so if you want to try interferon, talk to your doctor.
- **African Americans.** This ethnic group has a much lower response rate than the general population. Carroll Leevy, Sr., M.D., of the Sammy Davis Jr. Center near Newark, New Jersey, thinks that this may be in part because a larger proportion of African Americans than whites are genotype 1. But some people of all genotypes respond to interferon, so African Americans should still consider interferon therapy.

Interferon therapy presents special risks for people who have:

- **Bleeding varices,** a hepatitis complication in which delicate, swollen veins protrude from the inner walls of the esophagus and bleed easily.
- **Ascites,** a hepatitis complication in which fluid congregates in the chest, abdomen, and scrotal area, distending them.
- **Psychological problems** such as depression, anxiety, or confusion before starting interferon. Interferon can seriously worsen psychological problems, and confusion may make it difficult to take the drug properly.

If you have any of the above conditions and want to try interferon, ask your doctor about special opportunities such as experimental trials.

In addition, you will not be prescribed interferon if you:

- Are taking immunosuppressive drugs such as prednisone or cyclosporin after an organ transplant.
- Have an autoimmune disease such as lupus or diabetes.
- Suffer from kidney, lung, or heart disease.
- Are a child. Some young children who received interferon during clinical studies suffered a loss of appetite and retarded growth. Fortunately, children with hepatitis C have milder disease.

THE IRON FACTOR.   Iron deposits in the liver predict success with interferon as strongly as do viral genotype and the level of HCV in blood. Nine separate studies involving 434 people with HCV found that those with a large supply of iron in their livers were less likely to respond to interferon therapy. But those with no detectable iron were most likely to be complete responders.

AN "ACUTE" ISSUE.   A series of studies has offered evidence that interferon may help prevent acute infections from becoming entrenched and chronic. When patients with acute infections were given interferon for one to three months, both their ALT levels and HCV-PCR levels fell, although not to normal levels. Most maintained this improvement. Unfortunately, as we've seen, few people with HCV are diagnosed in the acute stage.

Interferon's Side Effects

The interferon didn't make me physically sick, just tired. But I am so depressed. I cannot take antidepressants because they bloat me so badly. I have tried them all—Prozac, Paxil, Zoloft, etc. So I cry a lot and I am on Ativan. That helps with anxiety, but I decided it is not enough. I'm seeing a therapist and she is sending me to a psychiatrist soon for a medication evaluation. And I'm looking for a support group. I need to meet people who have made it through this.

Dolores

Most people feel profoundly fatigued after taking interferon, especially at the beginning. Most people also have to contend with flulike symptoms—fever, chills, and muscle aches—that set in within eight hours of the first dose and persist for hours afterward. Strange as it seems, these symptoms are a good sign: Your fever and muscle aches are triggered by the release of your body's natural interferon and they mean that your body is fighting the virus.

Fortunately, the fatigue usually lightens after the first week. If possible, you should take your first few doses when you don't have to work, or if your doctor agrees, after work in the evenings. Build a nap or two into your daily routine, but don't give in to the temptation to become permanently affixed to your couch. Pursue some physical activity daily, because as you will read in Chapter 8, exercise helps maintain a healthy immune system. It also brightens your mood by producing endorphins, neurochemicals responsible for the famed "runner's high." Some people even find that moderate exercise relieves their fatigue.

Over-the-counter analgesics such as Tylenol or another brand of acetaminophen can relieve flulike symptoms. But ask your doctor what dose to take and don't overdo it: These OTC painkillers are metabolized by your liver, which doesn't need any additional stress.

Other common side effects of interferon therapy include nausea, irritability, depression, mild to moderate hair loss, and a loss of appetite. Most can be treated and all disappear after you stop treatment. Diarrhea and insomnia are less common side effects; you should tell your doctor about them. Let him or her know about *any* side effects that seem overwhelming or that suddenly worsen. Otherwise, try to roll with the punches. Try to eat smaller, more frequent meals. Remember that your hair will grow back after you stop taking interferon. And when battling side effects, don't forget to find out what works for others in your support group.

After a solid week of falling asleep just as the hands of my alarm clock crawled toward 5 A.M., I was exhausted, cranky, and depressed. My doctor had advised me to take sleeping aids only as a last resort, as they could strain my liver. Telma, a woman in my support group, asked, "How many cups of coffee do you drink?" I admitted I'd been drinking more to stay awake during the day. "Cut it out completely," she advised. "It's a vicious cycle. When I switched to decaf, I began sleeping better."

I went "cold turkey." It took a while, but now I sleep, not like a baby, but pretty darn well. My coworkers can live with me again.

Karen

Skin irritation can develop at the site where you inject interferon. To minimize this risk, your doctor will show you how to rotate injection sites. If it persists, call him or her to ensure that liver problems are not causing bruising.

Vitiligo, a patchy loss of skin color, often begins in small areas of the chest, arms, or face, then spreads. In most people, it progresses slowly or even reverses itself. This side effect can be treated.

Psychological side effects are quite common, but they lighten with time. Be prepared to experience sadness, depression, anxiety, and irritability, especially during the first few weeks. Here are some strategies for getting through that dangerous fortnight:

- Take interferon at night a few hours before bedtime; this can mute neuropsychiatric symptoms.
- Ask your physician for a referral to a psychiatric professional.
- Don't withdraw. You may be tempted to isolate yourself "until you feel better" but it is now that you need your friends. If they don't understand hepatitis C, do everyone a favor and educate them.

If your sadness doesn't go away, if it prevents you from working, or if it feels unbearable to you, be sure to tell your doctor, who may prescribe Prozac, Zoloft, or another antidepressant. Some can worsen liver damage.

People who are taking interferon may also experience **heart arrthymias** or an increase in **blood trigylcerides,** which your doctor will monitor or treat. **Kidney problems, optic neuritis,** and **rashes** are rare. Be sure to report signs and symptoms such as darkened urine, light stools, and any difficulty with your eyes to your doctor.

Red Flags: Certain side effects may constitute medical emergencies and you must contact your doctor *right away* if you experience them:

- Seizures, if you do not have a seizure disorder
- A high fever (above 102° F)
- A rash that spreads over much of your body
- Any sign of a bacterial infection, including, but not exclusively, fever, redness, pain, pus, skin breaks, or a red line extending from the site of an injection or injury
- Thoughts of suicide or homicide

Think twice before you give up on interferon because of side effects. Only 10 percent of patients actually discontinue the drug because they feel bad. This doesn't mean the other 90 percent are stronger than you. Maybe they found help. When you are having a problem with side effects, talk to your doctor, your nutritionist, and to everyone in your support group. Don't suffer in silence.

After Interferon

IF YOU DON'T RESPOND WELL TO INTERFERON: If you don't respond to interferon after the first course of therapy or are a partial responder, you must decide whether to undergo re-treatment.

A meta-analysis of 3,000 people suggested that many "non-responders" do respond to 5 million units of interferon thrice weekly for at least a year. Based on this research, most doctors have adopted these stronger, longer dosing schedules for interferon the second time around. Other "nonresponders" are helped by new, different forms of interferon such as Wellferon and Alferon.

Should you try re-treatment? That depends on why you didn't respond to the first course. Nonresponders with genotype 1 are likely to respond to re-treatment at higher doses and should pursue it. But because re-treatment involves a stronger dose of interferon for a longer period, it may not be a viable option if side effects contributed to your failure to respond. If you had to stop interferon therapy early because of side effects, you probably won't tolerate re-treatment unless the side effects can be lessened or better managed.

IF YOU ENJOY A SUSTAINED RESPONSE TO INTERFERON: If you have not relapsed after three years, congratulations on an excellent outcome: You may have banished the HCV from your blood and permanently arrested damage to your liver. But it is possible to relapse even after many years, and, unfortunately, most responders eventually relapse.

So it is very important to see your doctor regularly for tests, because only elevated ALT levels will warn you that it is time to undergo re-treatment.

IF YOU RELAPSE AFTER INITIALLY RESPONDING: If you relapse, you have plenty of company. But because you have previously responded to interferon, your chances of successful re-treatment are good. Combination treatment now offers a brighter hope for sustained response.

Combination Therapy

This approach marries interferon with one or more other agents in a medication "cocktail." Combination therapy illustrates the medical concept of *synergy*—a whole that is greater than the sum of its parts.

Interferon eliminates HCV in 15 percent of patients. Ribavirin is an agent that doesn't affect HCV at all. But when given with interferon, initial studies showed that ribavirin doubled interferon's response rate in most studies. Earlier this year the FDA approved Rebetron, a thrice-weekly combination of 500- to 600-milligram ribavirin capsules and 3-milligram interferon injections.

> I'm on Rebetron and I'm responding beautifully. I started six weeks ago, and my viral load has already dropped dramatically. But I'm having side effects. My blood cells are falling and so is my energy level. Nausea, fatigue, the works. My hair is dry and it's thinning. In a way that is the worst, because I've always been proud of my thick red hair. I have to keep reminding myself that it will come back. So I'm sticking with it. I have fear, but I'm determined that it'll work.
>
> Tamara

Tamara has good reason to stick with it. A recent *New England Journal of Medicine* study of 912 people with HCV showed that taking Rebetron is more effective than interferon for first-time users. After twelve months, combination therapy cleared the virus in 38 percent of patients—three times as many as in the interferon-only group! Viral levels remained undetectable for several months after the treatment was completed. A slew of similar studies have yielded the same results.

For those who have relapsed, Rebetron offers even more dramatic hope. It nearly eliminated the virus from the blood of half such patients, compared to a mere 5 percent of patients in relapse who took interferon alone. Rebetron boosted the rate of response by 500 percent!

SIDE EFFECTS. A meta-analysis involving 186 patients published in *Hepatology* presented more good news: The combination therapy enhances the effect of interferon without worsening its side effects. Like interferon taken solo, Rebetron may cause depression and flulike symptoms. It also caused anemia in one of every ten patients. Ribavirin can cause birth defects, so you should not begin Rebetron therapy if you plan to become pregnant.

Other Combination Therapies

At the June 1999 American Association for the Study of Liver Diseases conference, Michael Shiffman of the Medical College of Virginia unveiled a new form of interferon—**pegylated interferon alpha-2A,** or **PEG.** In a study of 159 patients with genotype 1, adding PEG to interferon allowed them to inject themselves only once a week and have response rates that were as good as Rebetron's and with fewer side effects than interferon alone.

Thymosin has also shown promise when used with interferon. In a sizable double-blind NIH trial of 110 patients, interferon reduced ALT levels to normal in 17 percent of patients. Levels fell in only 3 percent of those taking a placebo. But 42 percent of those taking a combination of thymosin and interferon achieved normal ALT levels. A 1996 study published in the journal *Gastroenterology* strongly suggested that **amantadine** holds similar promise. Both drugs are still years from your pharmacist's shelf, but you may be able to get them as part of a clinical trial.

Other Interferon-Based Treatment Strategies

CUSTOM-TAILORED DRUG REGIMENS.   As we have seen, different genotypes respond to different interferons. A key to successful treatment may be tailoring specific interferons to specific genotypic combinations, amount of virus in the blood, mode of infection, and other variables.

HIT THE HIV INFECTION HARDER.   That's the key to controlling HCV in people co-infected with HIV, according to joint research published by scientists at the Bar-Ilan University in Israel and the University of Illinois at Chicago in October 1998. "You want to treat the patients hard with drug therapy in the beginning and shut down production of the [HCV] virus," researcher Thomas Layden told *Science.* "This way you prevent drug-resistant mutations from developing."

The Israeli team used Intron to treat hepatitis C and used computers to model how quickly the virus spread in 23 patients.

They found that larger doses given early on could hamper viral growth within just two days.

Tips for Weathering Interferon Therapy

DON'T WAIT TO HYDRATE.   Unless your doctor has advised you to restrict your fluid intake, try drinking lots of water, especially around the time you give yourself a shot. Many swear that it eases symptoms.

VISIBLE MEANS OF SUPPORT.   At the risk of sounding like a broken record, I strongly urge you to join a support group. A support group is an invaluable source of tips for living with, managing, or even conquering side effects.

Even if no conventional medical treatment works for you, HCV probably never will become life-threatening or seriously compromise your quality of life. To maximize your chances of avoiding a serious complication, see your doctor regularly, so he or she can catch any signs of liver deterioration early, when it is easier to treat. The small percentage of people who develop liver cancer or severe cirrhosis must consider a transplant. See Chapter 10, "Extreme Remedies," for details.

On the Horizon

The following treatments are still in the planning or testing stage and have not been FDA-approved. But you may be able to obtain them by joining a clinical trial.

Earlier this year, 3M Company invested $400 million in clinical tests of **imiquimod**, as an oral antiviral treatment against hepatitis C. The FDA has already approved imiquimod in a cream for use on virus-caused genital warts, under the brand name Aldara. **N-acetylcysteine (NAC)** works as an antioxidant and reduces some blood concentrations of liver enzymes. NAC alone did not improve liver function in chronic hepatitis patients, but did enhance the effects of interferon. **Aspirin** and some other common over-the-counter pain relievers, called

NSAIDS (nonsteroidal anti-inflammatory drugs), also boosted liver function modestly, but only in small, ambiguous studies. So did the drugs pentoxyfylline and colchicine. These results must be duplicated in larger studies to gain any credibility. **Hydrophilic bile salts** seem to discourage many chronic inflammatory conditions involving the liver. One such agent, (tauro-)ursodeoxycholic acid, lowered serum ALT levels in recent study. **Cytokines,** chemicals that fine-tune the reactions of your immune system, are also undergoing limited trials. **Granulocyte-monocyte colony-stimulating factors (GM-CSFs)** have proved useful against some cancers, but have turned in a disappointing performance against hepatitis C: GM-CSFs proved expensive, ridden with side effects, and are far less effective than interferon. But if you are one of the few people who develops severe *neutropenia* during interferon therapy, GM-CSFs may help combat it so that you can finish your interferon course. **Protease inhibitors,** or PIs, a class of drugs that have proved very successful in slowing progression of HIV to AIDS, may work their magic against HCV within the next few years. Pharmaceutical companies are developing several PIs against key HCV enzymes. **Iron reduction** may be effective: N. Hayashi found that simply reducing the liver's iron content lowered ALTs to normal levels in half the patients he treated. A dozen studies involving 306 patients have confirmed his findings.

Where Is the HCV Vaccine?

A vaccine trains your immune system to defeat a dangerous virus. It teaches your immune system to "recognize" the virus and stimulates your immune cells to produce a militia of antibodies—living weapons that will destroy the virus immediately if it ever gains entry to your body.

A vaccine achieves all this using killed or inactivated *pieces* of a virus, for example, HCV, that cannot cause illness. The goal is to find a safe way to introduce such a fragment into the body so that the immune-system cells will recognize and manufacture defenses against the correct virus. You don't want to risk causing the disease you are trying to prevent, so the vaccine must be safely inactivated. Designing a vaccine against HCV will be challenging, because so far, HCV has proved too wily for us. HCV is a master of disguise, mutating so quickly that a candidate vaccine is quickly rendered worthless when it no longer "looks like" the virus.

Nevertheless, a vaccine *can* be designed: Vaccines have dispelled smallpox, polio, and other devastating diseases that we once perceived as incurable killers. The CDC estimates that it will be ten years before we see a vaccine for HCV, but this is because vaccine design will require that the government allocate resources and coordinate research efforts, something that has not happened yet.

Meanwhile, you *can* benefit from vaccination—against hepatitis A and B. You want to avoid co-infection with more than one hepatitis strain, which can lead to especially severe, quickly progressing liver disease.

By reading this book, you are becoming an informed medical consumer. But this information is no substitute for the care of a licensed physician. The only way to know how well you are doing is to obtain regular medical care and testing from a licensed physician and to carefully follow your doctor's advice.

For more information

Hepatitis Foundation International
30 Sunrise Terrace
Cedar Grove, NJ 07006
(800) 891-0707 or (201) 239-1035
Provides updated information on new diagnostic measures and treatments, referral to physicians, and access to a telecommunications network of patients with similar ailments.

The American Liver Foundation (ALF)
1425 Pompton Avenue
Cedar Grove, NJ 07009
(888) 4-HEPUSA or (973) 256-2550
www.alf.com

ALF will send you a variety of brochures and fact sheets covering all aspects of hepatitis C. ALF publishes *Progress,* a quarterly newsletter.

Hep C Connection

1741 Gaylord Street

Denver, CO 80206

This newsletter gives information about support groups, conferences, and recent research for hepatitis C patients. Call (303) 393-9395.

The American Holistic Medical Association

6728 Old McClean Village Drive

McClean, VA 22101

(703) 556-9728; fax: (703) 556-8729

E-mail: ahma@degnon.org

You can access the AHMA list of licensed physcians who have trained in a variety of complementary approaches for free online at www.holisticmedicine.org. Or you can mail $10 with a request for a hard copy.

Hepatitis and Liver Disease Referral Network

www.arens.com/hepnet/

This listing of hepatologists can assist your search for a physician.

Schering-Plough

www.hep-help.com

This Web site has information about the interferons manufactured by this company.

CHAPTER FIVE

Food: Dietary Armor for Your Immune System

One cannot think well, love well, sleep well, if one has not dined well.

—*Virginia Woolf,* A Room of One's Own

For a long time after I was diagnosed with hepatitis C, I felt tired and depressed. But mostly I felt victimized. I can't explain it, but one day I woke up and just had to *do* something. I made an appointment to see my doctor, and after we had talked about what I could do, changing my diet seemed a good place to start. Plus, I decided to try interferon, and she told me that eating the right foods could help. After talking to the dietitian, I had a battle plan.

I eats loads of fruits and vegetables, limit animal protein to five ounces daily, and I'm gradually replacing meat with beans, whole grains, and fish. I avoid salt and I force myself to drink water. I'm only up to five glasses a day, but I hate water, so that's progress. I don't drink alcohol at all.

I'm not cured, but I'm clearer-headed and I don't feel as tired as I used to. Now I feel optimistic that I can beat this, or at the very least head off serious liver damage. I'm in control again.

I feel good.

Nathalie

Good nutrition is an essential part of your strategy for living well with hepatitis C, and conventional and complementary practitioners alike acknowledge nutrition's key role in health and recovery. Departments of nutrition are firmly entrenched at medical institutions such as Harvard and Tufts, and schools of medicine increasingly require a course on nutrition.

Nutrition is especially important in promoting liver health, because the liver is the body's nutrient warehouse. It absorbs, processes, and stores essential nutrients, then releases them as the body needs fuel. Good nutrition helps you to defend your liver in two major ways: The right foods in the right forms ease the biological stress on this hardworking organ; and the right nutrients enhance the action of the immune system, which is fighting HCV and its effects.

This chapter provides invaluable information about nutrition. The right nutritional supplements for people with hepatitis C are described in Chapter 6, "Dietary Supplements," and their use is illustrated in Chapter 9, "Putting It All Together." The latter chapter provides examples of specific dietary strategies that have worked well for other people with hepatitis C. But the diet you follow must be prescribed or endorsed by your licensed physician, who may recommend a diet or dietary policy that differs from what is described here. Personal advice from your licensed physician always supersedes the more general information in this or any other book.

Eat for Health Maintenance

The right diet supports your overall health in several ways. It helps you to achieve or maintain a normal weight. It provides the right mix of proteins, carbohydrates, fats, fiber, vitamins, and minerals to keep your immune system operating at its peak. Vitamins and minerals are called micronutrients because they are needed in very small or trace amounts. A varied, balanced diet also provides other micronutrients and phytochemicals, necessary nutrients that are derived from plants. Scientists have not identified all the micronutrients we need for good health, so the only way to ensure you get enough is to eat lots of different kinds of foods.

As we saw in Chapter 1, your liver is the body's nutritional workhorse. It produces the bile that allows proper processing of fats and also metabolizes the protein and carbohydrates that provide energy for the body's maintenance and activities. The liver processes and stores many vitamins. Your liver rids the body of chemical pollutants, drugs, and poisons such as alcohol as well. To keep your liver operating at peak efficiency and to stave off cirrhosis as long as possible, you will need to maintain a normal weight and to avoid malnutrition.

You don't have to understand all the small details of the liver's metabolism, but you should be aware that the liver has two major metabolic pathways, called Phase I and Phase II. These are detoxification pathways—two major routes by which the liver purifies everything we take in and everything we produce. For example, acetaminophen compounds such as Tylenol are detoxified via Phase I; aspirin is detoxified via Phase II. You don't have to know which foods and drugs are eliminated by which pathway; such metabolic detail is beyond the scope of this work. But in order to clean and heal the liver, it is important to strengthen and stabilize both pathways, and that is why you must take in several foods, herbs, and supplements with the same functions.

As long as the liver is free of cirrhosis and fibrosis, you can probably absorb enough nutrients from a normal diet to support your liver and immune system. You can probably follow the same diet that is recommended by the United States Department of Agriculture (USDA) for healthy people without HCV, with just a few modifications if you are taking interferon.

This means you should eat a fiber-rich, predominately vegetarian diet that includes a lot of fruits, vegetables, and whole grains. You should eat relatively little sugar, meat, and fat.

The USDA recommends that you choose specific proportions of your diet from each of the five major food groups as illustrated by the United States Department of Agriculture, or USDA, dietary pyramid. It recommends six to eleven servings of grains, cereal, and pasta; three to five servings of vegetables;

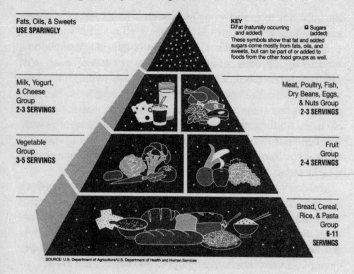

Fats, Oils, & Sweets
USE SPARINGLY

KEY
□ Fat (naturally occurring and added)   ◨ Sugars (added)
These symbols show that fat and added sugars come mostly from fats, oils, and sweets, but can be part of or added to foods from the other food groups as well.

Milk, Yogurt, & Cheese Group
2-3 SERVINGS

Meat, Poultry, Fish, Dry Beans, Eggs, & Nuts Group
2-3 SERVINGS

Vegetable Group
3-5 SERVINGS

Fruit Group
2-4 SERVINGS

Bread, Cereal, Rice, & Pasta Group
6-11 SERVINGS

SOURCE: U.S. Department of Agriculture/U.S. Department of Health and Human Services

Figure 3: *The USDA food pyramid*
United States Department of Agriculture

two to four servings of fruit; two to three servings from the milk, yogurt, and cheese group; and two to three servings of poultry, meat, or fish. The smaller number of servings is for people who consume about 1,600 calories a day, such as small sedentary women. The larger number is for those who consume about 2,800 calories a day, such as large active men. To sum up, the USDA recommends a high-fiber, low-fat diet that is plentiful in complex carbohydrates such as fruits, vegetables, and grains, and includes smaller amounts of fats and sugars.

If your diet is like that of most Americans, it doesn't resemble the USDA recommendations. Most people eat far too much fat, meat, sugar, and other simple carbohydrates and far too few vegetables, fruits, and whole grains. This is understandable, because many factors conspire to tempt us with quick, convenient, but not very healthy food choices.

Most adults work, leaving us with little inclination or time to plan and cook a carefully balanced meal after a busy day. Fewer families regularly sit down for dinners, further reducing the incentive to cook planned meals. Take-out and supermarket convenience foods such as microwaveable processed meals are tempting work- and time-savers. But they tend to be chock-full of fat, sugar, and preservatives and devoid of fresh produce. The advertising and packaging of processed convenience foods is also deceptive. For example, low-fat versions of foods tend to be very high in added sugar and salt. This means that in trying to improve your diet using processed foods, you can end up simply trading one bad dietary choice for another.

How can you eat a healthier diet? Use fewer processed foods. Instead, take just a little more time and effort to prepare fresh foods, so that you can control the amount of fat, sugar, salt, and other additions. This needn't take hours, because there are plenty of healthy shortcuts you can take. Let's look at some quick ways to improve your intake of each major food group:

GRAINS, CEREAL, AND PASTA. In general, the less-processed grain is better. Wheat berries are healthier than whole-grain bread, which is better than pasta. This means that you should shop with an eye to choosing minimally processed grains whenever possible. Eat oatmeal with oat bran, whole-grain toast, or low-fat organic granola instead of toasted white bread or sugary processed cereals for breakfast. Try substituting grains such as brown rice for potatoes. Try sprinkling wheat germ or miller's bran over other dishes; these will provide vitamins and fiber without changing the taste. Try tasty ethnic dishes that feature grains instead of a sandwich for lunch. Bulgur wheat salad, or tabouleh, is available in any health food store and in many supermarkets. Lentil salad or a low-fat version of spicy Jamaican beans and brown rice is another good-tasting source of unprocessed grains. To save time and effort, prepare large quantities of these dishes at once and freeze them.

VEGETABLES. Sulfur is an essential component of important proteins made by the liver. The high sulfur content in cruciferous vegetables such as broccoli, brussels sprouts, cabbage, and cauliflower makes them especially beneficial for the liver. So are garlic, beets, asparagus, and onions. These vegetables are especially potent cancer preventers as well. Bean sprouts are rich in chlorophyll, which cleanses the liver.

Fresh is best. If you can grow your own vegetables or buy at an organic market or from a farmers' market stand, you will get the best produce. Organic fare costs more, but some urban organic markets are cooperatives that will trade a few hours' work for a sizable discount on produce. If you are dependent upon supermarket fare, remember that their produce is likely to have sat in a warehouse before it sits on the supermarket shelves for a week or so. This is long enough to lose a good portion of the vitamins the veggies had when they were freshly picked, because some vitamins begin to disappear within hours. Also, supermarket produce is often genetically bred and chosen for its looks and its ability to resist spoilage when stored for long periods—not for its nutritive value or taste.

If you are on a tight budget and must use supermarkets, choose frozen vegetables and fruits with no preservatives. You will still risk pesticide exposure and will probably end up with vegetables that have lower levels of important nutrients and antioxidants. But many nutrients can survive freezing temperatures for weeks, so you will preserve the nutrients that are there. Many vegetables are frozen immediately after picking, so they may be even more nutritious than fresh produce that has been stored before sale. Frozen vegetables are also very convenient.

When preparing vegetables, remember that overcooking sabotages their nutritional value. Many vegetables are more nutritious when eaten raw or very lightly cooked. (Carrots are an exception: cooking them makes it easier for our bodies to extract their beta carotene.) So try eating more raw salads, and make a salad your main meal more often, because it's a great way to eat a wide variety of vegetables. Their inviting freshness and beautiful color make a dinner salad a nice change from a cooked main dish. Salads are also quick and easy to prepare. But don't overdo it; too much roughage can be as bad as too little if your liver infection is causing digestive problems, so ask your doctor or nutritionist how many raw greens and uncooked vegetables you should eat.

When you do cook vegetables, use as little heat as you can: Steaming them lightly preserves more of their taste, texture, appearance, and nutrients than boiling, baking, or sautéing them.

FRUITS. Fruits satisfy your desire for sweets while they provide cancer-fighting antioxidants and roughage that keeps your digestive system in good working order. Five fruits a day are easy if you begin thinking of fruits as guilt-free substitutes for cookies or potato chips. Lemons, limes, and grapefruits are especially good because they have a high nutrient-to-sugar ratio. But don't limit yourself to familiar treats such as citrus, apples, pears, and bananas. Explore less familiar fruits and hybrid fruits such as Asian pears, star fruits, guavas, persimmons, black currants, and tangelos.

MILK, YOGURT, AND CHEESE, COLLECTIVELY CALLED THE DAIRY GROUP. Milk poses a dilemma for many Americans. Dairy products are good sources of bone-strengthening calcium, and some dairy products are fortified with vitamin D. But Asians, African Americans, many Latinos—in fact, adults of most ethnic groups except for Caucasians—have high rates of lactose intolerance. Lactose intolerance is gastrointestinal distress in the form of bloating, cramping, and diarrhea that develops after a person drinks milk. It occurs because as children grow into adults, they often lose the ability to metabolize milk sugar.

Dairy products pose other problems for people with liver disease. The chemical structure of casein, the chief protein in milk, changes after pasteurization. It becomes more difficult to digest, which further strains the liver.

There are several solutions. Many lactose-intolerant people cannot drink milk, but can tolerate yogurt and cheese, which are sources of calcium. You also buy Lactaid brand milk and dairy products with the necessary enzyme added. Because milk is high in fat, try low-fat Lactaid milk or low-fat yogurt and cheeses. Milk's high fat content can create other problems for people with liver disease, too.

For calcium without the unwanted fats, try substitutes such as soy milk, rice milk, or oat milk. Soy milk is an especially good choice because it contains anticancer compounds. Canned salmon with the bones is another calcium-rich choice that also provides ample amounts of immune-enhancing omega-3 oils. Dark leafy greens such as collard greens also contain a moderate amount of calcium, although it is not as well absorbed by the body as the calcium in salmon and milk.

POULTRY, MEAT, AND FISH. This food group supplies high-quality protein and a variety of vitamins, especially B-complex vitamins. But meat can pose problems for people with hepatitis C as they develop cirrhosis. The proteins in red meat, ham, bacon, salami, and chicken are more easily converted to ammonia than are vegetable proteins. This means that proteins in these meats are more likely than vegetable protein to contribute to encephalopathy. You probably remember that encephalopathy is the forgetfulness and confusion that can result when someone with cirrhosis eats too much of the wrong sort of protein.

Beans, lentils, peas, fish, nuts, and seeds are better protein choices for people with hepatitis C. Use egg whites or egg substitutes such as Egg Beaters for protein without extra cholesterol. You already know that oily fish such as salmon, mackerel, and tuna give the added benefit of omega-3 oils that reduce your risks of artery and heart disease. But never eat raw fish or shellfish such as sushi or mussels; they can harbor toxins that target the liver and can be disastrous for someone whose liver is already weakened by HCV.

A word about condiments, salad dressings, and sauces: Get into the habit of reading the label before using them, because prepared dressings often derive their taste from high levels of salt, sugar, and fat. A teaspoonful of soy sauce is almost pure sodium, and ketchup is full of sugar and salt. Preparing your own condiments and salad dressings allows you to limit the content of harmful elements. If you choose to buy low-salt, low-fat, or low-sugar versions of condiments, exercise the same care as with other foods. Be sure to read the labels to make sure that you are not exchanging one unhealthy excess for another.

SODIUM. Sodium is the most important component of salt, and sodium is everywhere. Drinking water, food, condiments, even medications contain appreciable amounts of sodium. But it is salty eating choices that drive the sodium intake of the average American up to 6,900 milligrams a day. Sodium is everywhere in processed foods and condiments—as much as 1,000 milligrams in a single serving. The National Academy of Sciences says we need half that amount—500 milligrams a day—for health. In fact, the maximum safe intake is only 3,000 milligrams a day. That's a little more than one teaspoonful. The most you should consume is 5,000 milligrams a day, tops—that's about two teaspoonsful.

Because salt is an acquired taste, you can lose your "salt tooth" within a month, simply by eating less. Buy salt-free foods or, better yet, rely less on processed foods. See the next chapter, "Dietary Supplements," for more information on this mineral.

FAT. The USDA also says that no more than 30 percent of the total calories in your diet should come from fat—that's fat, saturated fat, and cholesterol combined. Fat constitutes 40 to 50 percent of the calories in most Americans' diets. But many experts feel that for disease prevention, even lower amounts of fat— 20 to 25 percent—are preferable, so you should consider 30 percent the upper limit of your dietary fat intake. See "Fats," on page 116, for a fuller discussion of dietary fats.

HOW LARGE IS A SERVING? The recommended serving sizes are smaller than you probably think. For example, one-half cup of cooked vegetables, one medium orange, or three ounces of cooked poultry or fish equal one serving.

GRAINS	VEGETABLES	FRUIT	DAIRY	PROTEIN
1 slice bread	½ cup cooked vegetables	1 medium banana	1 cup yogurt	½ cup cooked beans
½ cup cereal	1 cup raw vegetables	½ cup applesauce	1½ oz. cheese	1 egg
½ cup rice	¾ cup V-8 juice	¾ cup orange juice	1 cup milk	3 oz. cooked fish

For free information about portion sizes and nutritional content of a wide variety of foods, call the USDA at (202) 606-8000. Also see the resource list at the end of this chapter.

When Cirrhosis Develops

If you develop fibrosis or cirrhosis, your liver will have trouble completing all its nutritional tasks. This means that your nutritional needs will change, probably to a low-sodium, low-protein diet with several supplements. This chapter will explain your changing nutritional needs, and Chapter 6 explains how the right vitamin, mineral, and other nutritional supplements can help to delay liver damage and to compensate for the limitations of a damaged liver.

How Basic Nutritional Needs Change in Hepatitis C

WITH LITTLE OR NO CIRRHOSIS	TAKING INTERFERON	WITH CIRRHOSIS AND/OR LIVER CANCER
plant-based varied diet	plant-based varied diet	plant-based varied diet
NAS-recommended salt intake	NAS-recommended salt intake	restricted salt
USDA-recommended sugar intake	USDA-recommended sugar intake	USDA-recommended sugar intake

WITH LITTLE OR NO CIRRHOSIS	TAKING INTERFERON	WITH CIRRHOSIS AND/OR LIVER CANCER
USDA-recommended protein intake	possibly restricted protein	restricted protein
1 multivitamin, such as Rainbow Light's Just Once Iron-Free; vitamin D; vitamin E	additional vitamin and mineral supplements—see Chapter 6 for details	many special vitamin and mineral supplements—see Chapter 6 for details
USDA-recommended fat intake	USDA-recommended fat intake	fat supplements
USDA-recommended calorie intake	possible high-calorie supplements	possible high-calorie supplements
unlimited fluids	extra fluids	possibly restricted fluids

Food Additives

Because the liver must detoxify foods and substances in the body, it makes sense to avoid chemical additives and pesticide residues when you can. Shop in organic markets, try the organic section of the supermarket, or raise your own produce in a garden if you can. However, going organic is expensive and not everyone can afford to do it. On balance, it is much more important to avoid alcohol, maintain a normal weight, and eat a balanced, varied diet. If you don't buy organic foods, remember to thoroughly clean produce to minimize chemical residues and waxes.

Don't Wait to Hydrate

If you have no cirrhosis and your doctor has not restricted your fluid intake, drink at least eight glasses of water daily to help your liver and kidneys metabolize the drugs you are taking. But keep sugar- and caffeine-loaded beverages to a minimum. Many people prefer herbal teas because most have no caffeine, but before you stock up, be sure to read their labels and ask your doctor about them. Some, such as comfrey, can harm the liver; see the end of Chapter 7 for a discussion of these. **If you develop cirrhosis,** you may have to limit the fluids you take in to avoid *ascites* and loss of potassium.

Protein: A Balancing Act

Protein is essential to life. Egg whites, milk, fish, poultry, nuts, beans, and red meat are all sources of protein, which your pancreas breaks down into their constituent amino acids. These amino acids are absorbed through the intestine into the liver. In the liver, amino acids play a dual role—some are used for energy and others are put together to make new proteins. Your liver constructs more than a dozen proteins, each with a specific role in the body. *Albumin,* for example, makes up blood plasma; *ferritin* holds iron; *P-450* processes chemicals and drugs; *renin* maintains blood pressure; and *clotting factors* help the blood to clot normally.

Proteins are building blocks of muscle, so you must eat enough to avoid muscle wasting and profound fatigue. This is especially vital if you are taking interferon, which often causes fatigue. But in people with impaired liver function, too much protein can also cause problems such as fatigue and *encephalopathy,* a mental condition marked by forgetfulness, confusion, personality change, and even coma. **If you develop cirrhosis,** getting the right amount of protein becomes very tricky. Damaged livers allow blood levels of ammonia, a toxic by-product of protein metabolism, to rise, and excess ammonia can cause encephalopathy. Scientists think that ingesting more aromatic (circular) amino acids than amino acids that are arranged in branched chains may encourage encephalopathy. So, as we saw earlier, your doctor may recommend a vegetarian diet, because vegetable proteins contain fewer aromatic amino acids. Definitely avoid ham, bacon, beef, chicken, salami, buttermilk, and gelatin, because their amino acids are very easily turned into ammonia. Your doctor or nutritional advisor may recommend a supplement drink with a preponderance of branched-chain amino acids. Or you may be treated with a diet that is quite low in protein—from 25 to 60 grams a day.

Carbohydrates

Carbohydrates are either *simple,* such as those found in table sugar and most fruits, or *complex,* found in breads, beans, rice and other grains, cereals, pasta, and vegetables. You should choose mostly high-fiber complex carbohydrates such as whole grains. Eat smaller amounts of simple sugars. The liver processes and stores carbohydrates as *glycogen,* then releases the precise amount of glycogen the muscles need for fuel. Complex carbohydrates, also called starches, provide healthy, sustained levels of energy. They also provide more beneficial fiber. **If you develop cirrhosis,** it becomes even more important to choose complex carbohydrates, because they do not trigger extreme blood-sugar highs (hyperglycemia) and lows (hypoglycemia) that can affect an impaired liver called on to process simple sugars.

Artificial Sweeteners

If your doctor, registered dietitian, or nutritional counselor advises you to eat less or to avoid table sugar, your first reaction may be reach for the Sweet 'n' Low, Equal, or another artificial sweetener. In general, this is a bad idea. Some sugar substitutes, such as xylitol, are nutritive, and your body metabolizes them similarly to sugar. But other nonnutritive sweeteners, such as aspartame and saccharin, do not disturb blood sugar or add weight but do remain shadowed by health questions. Many artificial sweeteners seem to trigger a craving for sweets, which certainly defeats the purpose of a sugar substitute. Another, less common, type of sugar substitute, called L-sugar, tastes like sugar, but is not metabolized by the body because it is the chemical "mirror image" of the sugar we stir into our coffee. The label lists a sugar beginning with the prefix "l-," such as "l-dextrose." L-sugars are excreted unused, have no calories, and don't affect the blood sugar. But they do cause intestinal upset and diarrhea that leaches precious vitamins and minerals from the body. So they are not a good choice for the person with hepatitis C, who needs to retain as many nutrients as possible.

Foods and beverages naturally sweetened with very small amounts of licorice, fructose, or honey are better options.

Fats

> I'm from the South, so is my husband, and we believe in frying. Breakfast was always something like ham, buttered grits, fried eggs, home fries . . . well, you get the picture. When my doctor told me I had to stop cooking with fat and try to eat a mostly vegetarian diet, he might as well have told me to fly home: I couldn't imagine how I would do such a thing. Thank goodness for Betty, his dietitian. She showed me little tricks like making omelets with egg whites and Pam, substituting smoked turkey for pork, and using lemon juice instead of salt. She also encouraged me to try different fresh fruits and vegetables. Well, to make a long story short, that was a year ago, my liver enzymes are down, and my swollen stomach and legs look normal again. I have more energy and I'm much happier with the way I look. Now the thought of a greasy, salty breakfast nauseates me!
>
> Letitia

The average American eats too much fat. A high-fat diet contributes to many serious health problems, including heart disease, stroke, and some cancers. Fat has 9 calories per gram, more than twice as much as that in carbohydrates and protein, so fat contributes to our national girth as well. The USDA recommends that you take in no more than 30 percent of your calories from fats. Even less—20 to 25 percent—seems to protect against many diseases, including cancers. But don't eat less than 20 percent of your calories from fat unless you doctor specifically advises you to, because fat is also important to maintaining proper metabolism and weight.

You must also eat the right kind of fats. Consuming too many saturated fats dangerously increases dietary cholesterol; so does eating food with high cholesterol levels, such as eggs and pork.

Polyunsaturated fats have been implicated in cancer. Mono-unsaturated fats, such as abound in olive oil, and foods rich in omega-3 oils (described below) are better choices.

Fats are very important in managing your hepatitis C. The liver processes triglycerides, fat precursors that we obtain from oils, butter, dairy foods, and meat, to produce energy. The liver also secretes bile, which is necessary to transform triglycerides into a water-soluble form that can be carried by the blood to sites where it is needed for energy. The liver produces the body's stores of cholesterol as well. **If you develop cirrhosis,** the liver loses function and cholesterol production drops. Cholesterol is the nutritional "bad guy" implicated in hardening of the arteries (atherosclerosis), stroke, and heart disease, but it is also an essential component of body tissues such as collagen: We need some cholesterol to survive.

If the cirrhotic liver cannot produce enough bile to adequately digest fat, the fat is excreted in the stool, a condition called *steatorrhea,* which makes your stool light-colored. Or it is stored in visible deposits on the liver, a condition called *fatty liver.* If either develops, you should reduce your fat intake to 40 to 70 grams daily. Omega-3 oils are naturally occurring fatty acids that lower cholesterol levels and discourage blood vessel damage. In controlled studies, people who ate diets rich in these fatty acids had less artery-clogging cholesterol in their bloodstreams, and so were at lower risk for stroke, heart disease, and other serious ailments. Preserving the health and function of the blood vessels that supply the liver is very important for people with hepatitis C. Eating fatty fish such as salmon and mackerel three times a week produces the desired cholesterol-lowering effect.

Fat substitutes such as olestra, marketed as Simplesse, provide the satisfying taste and texture we crave with no calories and no fat. But olestra leaches fat-soluble vitamins such as A and K from the body. People with cirrhosis are already deficient in these vitamins, so this is an unacceptable price to pay for fat-free noshing. Also, 20 percent of people who eat chips, ice cream, and other treats made with these substitutes experience gastrointestinal problems that include cramping and diarrhea.

Eat to Minimize Interferon's Side Effects

We saw in Chapter 4 that interferon can cause flulike symptoms, fatigue, anxiety, nausea, diarrhea, and appetite loss leading to weight loss. Eating correctly can ease these symptoms.

FOR NAUSEA. Eating smaller, more frequent meals helps many people. High-calorie supplements such as Ensure and Suplena are appropriate for some people and are discussed in the next chapter.

FOR FATIGUE. Your nutritionist, registered dietitian, and doctor will work with you to choose the right balance of complex carbohydrates and protein for sustained energy.

FOR ANXIETY. Caffeine makes anxiety worse and interferes with sleeping. If you have these problems, consider switching to decaffeinated coffee or eliminating coffee and tea altogether. To "taper off," and perhaps avoid the headachy symptoms of caffeine withdrawal, add increasing amounts of decaf to your favorite coffee. Drink lots of water instead; many people swear that this softens interferon's side effects.

FOR DEPRESSION. Depression can't be banished by a single good meal, but setting the stage for a pleasant dining experience can help. Take a tip from good restaurants and make presentation an art: You don't have to save the good china, silver, candlesticks, and soft music for guests; treat yourself sometimes! Prepare your favorite foods more often. Forbid arguing, discipline, or discussions of money problems at the table, and turn the news programs off during the dinner hour.

Some foods can directly worsen your mood. Too much sugar can lower insulin in a rebound effect, which can put you in a blue mood. Alcohol's high is often followed by depression and sleep disorders, not mention profound liver damage. Mixing sugar and aspartame, the artificial sweetener found in Equal, induces psychological changes in some people.

Juice Fasts

Fasting can help to eliminate the body's entrenched toxins. When juices are taken during the fast, they can provide a quick infusion of vitamins and minerals that help fight infection. Because little energy is required to digest juices, they can supply enough energy over short periods, but fasting should be undertaken during warm weather. Otherwise, the calories the body uses to maintain its metabolism during cold weather may sap needed energy. Juices supply no fiber, so they should not be considered complete fruits, and you should not routinely substitute them for fruit in your diet unless your doctor specifically tells you to. Diabetics and pregnant or lactating women should not undertake fasts.

In contrast, plain-water fasting is not recommended for people with hepatitis C, because often their chronic loss of appetite can make it hard for them to absorb adequate nutrition, and a prolonged period without any food and drink can further upset their already disturbed metabolic balance and digestion.

But a two- to five-day juice fast can help relieve the gastrointestinal problems that plague some people with hepatitis C, says Kenneth B. Singleton, M.D., MPH. He suggests raw unprocessed organic beet, carrot, or celery juices. If you use beet juice, dilute it with water in a one-to-one ratio to reduce its sugar content. For other juice-fast recipes, read *The Complete Book of Juicing* by M. Murray (Prima Publishing, 1992).

Get Expert Advice

As liver disease progresses, your nutritional needs may become increasingly complex and you will need professional help. Your doctor may refer you to a registered dietitian or nutritionist who will monitor you for nutritional deficiencies and change your diet as your liver health changes. Registered dietitians must undergo training and certification, and you can find a qualified dietitian in your area by calling the American Dietetic Association National Referral Line at 1-800-366-1655.

But in most states, a person can call himself a nutritionist whether he is a highly trained, experienced professional or not. To protect yourself, ask about the person's qualifications, or better yet, ask your doctor for a referral.

Remember that, as was discussed in Chapter 4, your doctor coordinates all your care. Make sure that she is aware that you are obtaining dietary advice, and do not follow the advice of a nutritional counselor if it conflicts with anything your doctor advises.

Maintain a Normal Weight

The USDA Department of Nutrition recommends that you take in 1,500 to 2,800 calories daily depending upon your gender, size, age, metabolism, and energy level. Smaller, less active women should ingest fewer calories, and larger, more active men should gravitate toward the higher caloric end.

Interferon therapy or cirrhosis makes some people nauseous after taking just a few forkfuls of food, so taking in enough calories may become difficult. If you are overweight, you may welcome this side effect, but you need to be well nourished to fight HCV complications, so this is usually not the time to go on a diet. However, if you are obese, that is, if you weigh at least 20 percent more than you should, your doctor may suggest that you manage your weight, because obesity can hinder your immune response and it is also a risk factor for infection.

Avoid Alcohol

Your liver must work overtime to metabolize alcohol, and a liver infected by HCV does not need the extra biological stress. Alcohol can also cause fatty liver, which impedes its function. The most credible studies indicate that drinking more than 30 grams of alcohol a day—that's one glass of wine or one can of beer daily—can injure a liver with hepatitis. But there is no proven safe level of alcohol intake for a person with HCV, so many clinicians tell HCV patients without cirrhosis or fibrosis that they may drink only "occasionally." If you develop cirrhosis, drinking alcohol is out of the question.

I used to be an oenophile: Wine was my hobby. My wife and I spent holidays in the wine country of several states, and I went to tastings at least once a month. When I learned I had hepatitis C, I gave the contents of my cellar to my synagogue for its annual auction. Now I don't drink at all. Instead, we've taken up golf and we vacation at beautiful courses. I miss wine, but not as much as I would miss my liver!

Dan

If you develop cirrhosis and continue to drink, you must accept that your drinking is beyond your control and ask your doctor for help. Some doctors prescribe the vitamins thiamin and folic acid for people who drink heavily, but this is a stopgap measure at best. If you don't stop drinking, you will face accelerated cirrhosis and a higher risk of liver cancer—problems far worse than a vitamin deficiency.

This chapter has explained why eating the right foods is an important strategy for managing your hepatitis C. But there's more to your nutritional campaign—supplements can help, too. Chapter 6 explains how.

For more information

Bibliography

Ballantine, Rudolph. *Transition to Vegetarianism.* Himalaya Publishers, 1987.

Fugh-Berman, Adriane, M.D. "Dietary Supplements and Nutrition." In *Alternative Therapies: What Works.* William & Wilkins, 1997.

Washington, Harriet A. "The Vitamin Revolution." *Health* magazine, August 1998. Reprinted in *Women's Health Guide 2000.* Editor John Poppy © 2000 Time, Inc. Health "Superfoods" Editor John Poppy, © 1999 Time Health Media.

Online Sources

Intelihealth
www.intelihealth.com/
This Johns Hopkins University site provides low-fat, low-sodium

versions of recipes. It also displays nutrition-label information for a wide assortment of foods by brand name.

Organizations

The American Association of Naturopathic Physicians

2366 Eastlake Avenue, Suite 322

Seattle, WA 98102

(206) 323-7610

Provides help in finding a dietician.

USDA Center for Nutrition Policy and Promotion

1120 20th Street, NW, Suite 200, North Lobby

Washington, DC 20036

(202) 606-8000

Web site: usda.gov/cnpp

This organization publishes *Dietary Guidelines for Americans*. Write or go online for detailed, readable, and free USDA publications on basic nutrition, but be warned: These tend to be conservative on the issues of vitamins and supplements.

The American Institute for Cancer Research

(800) 843-8114

Distributes free newsletters, pamphlets, and practical tips on good nutrition. Its toll-free nutrition hot line is staffed by a registered dietitian.

Vegetarian Resource Group

P.O. Box 1463

Baltimore, MD 21203

(410) 366-8343

Provides information about vegetarianism.

CHAPTER SIX

Dietary Supplements

Many doctors still insist that taking supplements of vitamins, minerals, and other nutrients is unnecessary if one eats a well-balanced diet. But even for the relatively few Americans who actually consume that well-balanced diet, some supplements are usually necessary to meet National Academy of Sciences, or NAS, guidelines. As we saw in Chapter 5, healthy people need take only one multivitamin tablet, one serving of folic-acid-fortified bread or cereal or a 400-microgram folic acid supplement, and one 600 to 800 IU vitamin E supplement a day as dietary insurance.

But most NAS standards were designed to prevent deficiency disease, not to maximize wellness. And they don't always meet this modest goal. For example, when vitamin-D expert Michael Holick studied 290 people at Boston University Medical Center in 1998, he found that 46 percent of those who took multi-vitamins had deficient vitamin-D blood levels. The USDA reports that fewer than 70 percent of Americans consume the recommended daily allowance for calcium and magnesium as well as A, B-complex, and C vitamins.

Supplements That Treat Hepatitis

People with hepatitis C must do more than avoid deficiency. If a person with little or no liver damage takes the right vitamins and minerals in doses higher than the RDA (recommended daily allowance), he or she can foster a high state of wellness and protect against disease. Supplements do this by enhancing the efficiency of the immune system, which is key to limiting liver damage and to preventing the progression of cancer. Also, the antioxidant action of some supplements limits liver tissue destruction and cancerous changes in the liver.

This means that people without cirrhosis should not wait to enhance their nutrition: They should consider carefully selected supplements to avoid weight loss, boost immune-system functioning, discourage cirrhosis, and protect against cancer. Some physicians simply recommend two over-the-counter multivitamin tablets for patients without cirrhosis, but this is not a good idea. Two multivitamins supply large doses of some vitamins and minerals that can harm people with hepatitis C, such as niacin and iron. People with hepatitis C who do not have fibrosis or seriously elevated liver enzymes should take a daily multivitamin, up to 800 IU of vitamin E, 400 to 600 IU of vitamin D, and one serving of folic-acid-fortified bread or cereal. Once liver damage sets in, you will need additional supplements, as explained in this chapter and as prescribed by your physician.

First, here are the nutrients people with hepatitis C should look for in a once-daily multivitamin. Choose one that is food-based and that does not contain iron, such as Rainbow Light Just Once Iron-Free.

VITAMINS

Micronutrient	Dose
Vitamin A (as beta-carotene)	5,000–10,000 IU
Vitamin C	200–500 mg
Vitamin D	100 IU; 400 IU if you don't take a separate vitamin D supplement

Micronutrient	Dose
Vitamin E (natural)	60–120 IU
Vitamin K	30–90 mcg
Vitamin B$_1$ (thiamin)	6 mg
Vitamin B$_2$ (riboflavin)	6 mg
Vitamin B$_3$ (niacinamide)	no more than 30 mg; 20 is preferable
Vitamin B$_6$ (pyroxidine)	6 mg
Folic Acid	400 mcg
Vitamin B$_{12}$ (cyanocobalamin)	25 mcg
Biotin	300 mcg
Pantothenic acid	30 mg

MINERALS

Micronutrient	Dose
Calcium	30 mg
Iodine	100 mcg
Magnesium	30 mg
Zinc	5 mg
Selenium	25–75 mcg
Copper	0.5–2.0 mg
Manganese	no more than 2.5 mg
Chromium	50–100 mcg
Molybdenum	12–1,000 mcg
Potassium	20–400 mg (potassium is optional; if you need it, your doctor will prescribe a supplement or food source)
Boron	50 mcg (this is optional and no daily requirement has been established)
Vanadium	8 mcg (this is optional and no daily requirement has been established)

OTHER MICRONUTRIENTS

(These are optional; you can take them in separate supplements if you need them.)

Micronutrient	Dose
Bioflavonoids	60 mg or more
Choline	15 mg or more
Inositol	15 mg or more
PABA	5 mg or more
Proteases	source and dose varies
Amylases	source and dose varies
Spirulina	source and dose varies

Many vitamins offer a small amount of a few herbal extracts, which is acceptable, if you tell your herbalist you are taking them. But don't choose a vitamin that offers a large amount of or a large number of herbal extracts. Your herbalist may recommend specific amounts of certain herbs, and large amounts in the multivitamin may throw off the dose or may even introduce an herb with a competing action.

A person who is taking interferon, or has developed cirrhosis or liver cancer, may also need special high-calorie supplements that can counter the treatment-related nausea and fatigue that sabotages good nutrition.

If you develop cirrhosis, you will need extra nutrients because you may not be able to absorb and process vitamins, minerals, proteins, and fats from food or from ordinary vitamin pills. Special, easily absorbed supplements such as MCT oil and protein supplements can save the day.

But supplements must be used with respect. As we saw in the last chapter, the wrong supplement or an overdose of the right one can have a paradoxical effect. For example, normal protein intake maintains muscle in people without liver damage, but people with cirrhosis should limit protein.

I have not suffered any significant liver damage and I want to keep it that way. So I went to the health food store and asked the clerk what supplements were good for hepatitis. I came home with seventy dollars' worth of supplements. After two weeks, I didn't see any difference except a yellowish tinge to my skin. I was afraid that I was developing jaundice. I called my doctor's office. "You've wasted most of your seventy dollars," Rashida, the nutritionist, said, then explained that although the 400-milligram vitamin C pills would help my liver, the omega-3 oil supplements were ineffective and the iron pills could be dangerous to someone with hepatitis C! Fortunately, the "jaundice" turned out to be harmless yellow coloring from the beta-carotene pills I'd bought. "Next time, call me *before* you go shopping for supplements," said Rashida. "I'll guide you to the right ones; that's why I'm here."

Frank

To avoid the dangers of overdose or unforeseen side effects, do not take vitamins or minerals unless they are prescribed by your doctor or recommended by your registered dietitian. Many vitamins and minerals act in concert, and taking too much of one can induce a deficiency in another. So don't assume that if a small amount is good, a larger amount must be better. As you have read above, many vitamins can help or hinder your liver, depending on their dose. Overdoses can be serious, even life-threatening. Choose food-derived supplements without fillers, starches, colorings, and yeast to minimize the possibility of allergic reactions.

VITAMINS

Vitamins are chemicals that are necessary to life. Our bodies cannot make sufficient quantities of most vitamins, so we obtain them from food or supplements in very tiny amounts. We divide vitamins into those that are soluble in water and the fat-soluble group. The necessary amounts of the water-soluble B-complex and C vitamins are measured in grams (g), milligrams (mg), and micrograms (mcg). Grams are one thousand times larger than milligrams, and milligrams are a thousand times larger than micrograms. To put these amounts in perspective, consider that a teaspoon holds 2 grams of salt: That's 2,000 milligrams or 2,000,000 micrograms. International units (IU) are used to measure the fat-soluble antioxidant vitamins A, D, E, and K.

Antioxidant is a term that is often used and seldom defined. To explain its meaning, I will define a few other terms. *Oxidation* is a chemical change that can weaken and distort materials. For example, oxidized iron is rust. Oxidized blood-vessel walls are scarred and rigid with atherosclerosis. Oxidized cells in liver tissue are prone to cirrhosis and cancer. The substances that promote this oxidation are called *oxidants*. A *free radical* is a prime example of an oxidant. It is an incomplete, chemically unstable molecule. Free radicals career from cell to cell, injuring each one they touch, like a pugnacious drunk at a concert. Antioxidants are the bouncers: They chemically "link arms" with the free radical, escorting it from the scene. Antioxidants protect cells against corrosive changes that can lead to tissue injury and cancer. Many vitamins function as antioxidants.

PARADOXICAL EFFECTS OF VITAMINS. People with hepatitis C often need supplements as their liver disease progresses, and these supplements can significantly benefit their health. What's more, the right vitamins will not further injure the liver, as pharmaceuticals can. But it is important to use carefully chosen therapeutic doses of the right supplements with the aid of your nutritionist or dietitian and physician. You should also realize that more is not always better. Large doses of vitamins sometimes have a paradoxical effect, that is, a large dose seems to *cause* the damage that a smaller dose discourages. For example, vitamin D helps protect bones in therapeutic doses. But an overdose erodes bone. Similarly, vitamin C's antioxidant action protects against cancer in doses below 500 milligrams daily. But higher doses are associated with higher cancer risks. This is because at high doses vitamin C can cease to be an antioxidant and become an oxidant, encouraging the very tissue damage it usually prevents. Some professionals do prescribe larger doses of vitamin C, explaining that they can safely do so because they balance the vitamin with other beneficial supplements that counter its oxidative nature.

The take-home message? Megadoses of vitamins sometimes improve your health, but be sure to work with a professional in determining the amounts of vitamins and minerals you need.

Vitamin A

Vitamin A keeps your skin, hair, and nails strong and beautiful. It maintains healthy bones, glands, and gums. Vitamin A is also key to good vision: A deficiency causes night blindness, and if it lasts long enough, complete blindness, although the latter is very rare. Beta-carotene is the form of vitamin A found in produce such as cantaloupe, carrots, and broccoli. Leafy green and yellow vegetables are also excellent sources of beta-carotene. Vitamin A fights infection and beta-carotene increases the body's levels of cancer-fighting antibodies, T-cells, and natural killer cells. Vitamin A supports thymus gland function as well, and that gland is crucial in the prevention and treatment of cancer.

Vitamin A occurs naturally (as beta-carotene) in carrots and many other vegetables, fish, and animal foods. Cirrhosis causes a deficiency.

Too much vitamin A leads to liver toxicity; so can too much retinoic acid, a related molecule. Because such overdoses of vitamins A and D are especially dangerous to people with hepatitis C, choose beta-carotene instead; excess beta-carotene is excreted, so it is impossible to overdose.

It is better to get your A from food than from a pill. But if liver damage prevents vitamin A absorption, your doctor may recommend that you take an easily absorbed liquid supplement.

BETA-CAROTENE SUPPLEMENT (supplies VITAMIN A)
What it does: Beta-carotene increases the body's levels of cancer-fighting antibodies, T-cells, and natural killer cells.
How it works: Our bodies turn beta-carotene into vitamin A, an antioxidant, with no chance of overdose.

Who this should benefit: People who can no longer absorb enough beta-carotene from their diets.

Who should avoid this: Two studies have linked beta-carotene supplements to higher cancer rates in smokers, and although no cause-and-effect relationship has been established, the jury is still out. It would be prudent for smokers to avoid beta-carotene supplements until more definitive studies are conducted.

Recommended formulation: Pills and liquid.

Usual dosage range: Between 15,000 and 30,000 IU (10 to 20 mg) daily.

Side effects: None reported.

Caveats: High doses of vitamin A can cause liver damage, which can result in jaundice. High doses of beta-carotene can also give a yellow cast to skin that is not jaundice but a safe, reversible deposit of beta-carotene. You must see your doctor to know which you have.

B Vitamins

B-complex vitamins include a whole constellation of vitamins that act in concert to bolster immunity and offer nutritional support to people with liver cancer. Many cancers are promoted by vitamin deficiencies. The B vitamins also ease depression and insomnia and help raise blood cell counts, which tend to fall during cancer and cancer treatment. Except where noted, B vitamins are primarily found in organ meats, seafood, poultry, fortified grains, cereals, and dairy products.

You should not take supplements of individual B vitamins, because B vitamins act in concert, and a large dose of one can induce a deficiency of another. *Thiamin* (B_1) helps digestion and nerve function. It seems to boost immunity and discourage cancers; some doctors give it to alcoholics, who are often deficient. *Riboflavin* (B_2) is needed to process foods and helps orchestrate the release of energy to cells. Riboflavin also helps maintain normal vision and is an essential component of tumor-fighting T- and B-cells. T-cells are immune-system components that are especially important in the body's defense against hepatitis C. *Niacin* (B_3) should be avoided because it is toxic to the liver.

Pyridoxine (B_6) helps direct protein and carbohydrate metabolism and helps form red blood cells. B_6 is also key to the production of immune-system proteins and cancer-fighting antibodies that slow or arrest tumor growth. *Cyanocobalamin* (B_{12}) is necessary for the construction of the genetic molecules DNA and RNA, and it also helps form red blood cells. B_{12} discourages cancer by "turning off" disorganized precancerous cells so that normal growth patterns can be restored. In some studies, administering B_{12} lengthened the survival time of people with cancers. *Folic acid* is another key player in DNA and RNA synthesis, and red blood cell formation, and it also prevents neural-tube birth defects. It supports the immune system and prevents derangement of the DNA in healthy cells, which in turn prevents cancerous changes. Too little folic acid causes weight loss and anemia, and the law requires that it be added to most cereals and breads. An Argentinian study suggests that folic acid, vitamin B_{12}, and vitamin C may help to restore the skin color of people who develop vitiligo, which affects some people on interferon therapy.

Pantothenic acid (B_5) is necessary to the manufacture of hormones and other chemicals that control nervous-system function. It also bolsters the immune system. It is found in nearly all foods, and we also produce some with the help of intestinal bacteria. *Biotin* is produced by intestinal bacteria and can be gleaned from meats, fish, vegetables, and seeds. Biotin helps to process glucose and to make fatty acids. Cirrhosis causes B-vitamin deficiency.

B-COMPLEX VITAMIN SUPPLEMENTS.

B-complex supplements consist of folic acid with vitamin B_{12} and sometimes one or more of B_1, B_2, or B_6. B-complex formulations often contain vitamin C.

What it does: May protect against cancer, including liver cancer; helps delay progression to cirrhosis and cancer; sometimes restores skin color to people who develop vitiligo as a side effect of interferon therapy.

How it works: Provides folic acid in balance with other water-soluble vitamins.

Who this should benefit: People without significant liver damage; people with vitiligo, which was discussed in Chapter 4.

Who should avoid this: People with seizure disorders and cancer; see "Caveats."

Recommended formulation: Take B vitamins in the combination that your dietitian recommends for your level of liver health. Don't take a single B-vitamin supplement, because they must be used in balanced formulations: Too high a dose of one can cause a "rebound" deficiency of another. B_{12} can be injected under the tongue or sprayed into a nostril if liver damage prevents absorbing enough through the gut. The B-complex vitamin niacin is toxic to the liver, especially the sustained-release form.

Usual dosage range: 300+ mg of folic acid; between 10 and 100 mg each of B_1 B_2, and B_3; up to 50 mg of B_6; 50 to 100 mcg of B_{12}, and up to 500 mg of C daily.

Side effects: Too much folic acid can cause nervous-system damage and can mask a B_{12} deficiency; folic acid can also block absorption of zinc. Prolonged very high levels of C promote cancer and tissue damage.

Caveats: Do not take folic acid if you are taking certain anti-convulsive or chemotherapy drugs, among them phenytoin, methotrexate, colchicine, and trimethoprim. They work by depressing folic acid levels.

Vitamin C

Vitamin C, or *ascorbic acid,* is extremely useful for people with hepatitis C because it strengthens blood vessel walls, which can help discourage dangerous bleeding in people with esophageal varices. Some practitioners inject vitamin C to bolster the immune response of patients with hepatitis C and discourage cancer.

Vitamin C is an antioxidant that protects against cancer and tissue damage. Most citrus fruits, cabbage, broccoli, peppers, and plantains are rich in vitamin C. Nobel laureate Linus Pauling did much to popularize C when he claimed that very large doses of C cure everything from cancer to the common cold. But high levels can cause kidney stones and diarrhea, and both problems are more common in people with hepatitis C.

Even worse, medical reports suggest that vitamin C can have a Jekyll-and-Hyde character. If you suddenly fall back to normal levels after taking high levels for prolonged periods, you may develop symptoms of deficiency disease—scurvy—in a rebound effect. At high doses, vitamin C can act as an oxidant, promoting tissue damage and cancer rather than discouraging them. In fact, doses greater than 500 milligrams daily are associated with higher cancer risks. Vitamin C's negative effects are worsened if you have large stores of iron in your body (see the discussion of iron on page 139).

VITAMIN C (ascorbic acid) SUPPLEMENT

What it does: Neutralizes carcinogens, preserves tissue health, maintains strong blood vessel walls.

How it works: Antioxidant action delays cancer and tissue damage; vitamin C also enhances the antioxidant action of vitamins A and E. But at high levels, C may *promote* tissue damage and cancer.

Who this should benefit: People at most stages of hepatitis C. Vitamin C delays or prevents liver tissue damage, including cirrhosis and cancer.

Who should avoid this: In people with high blood levels of iron, Vitamin C triggers a dangerous flood of iron into the bloodstream, so have your iron levels tested first if you are considering taking a supplement. People with advanced liver cancer should also avoid vitamin C supplements.

Recommended formulation: Pills and capsules, and injection by physicians.

Usual dosage range: 200 mg a day, but no more than 500 mg daily if you are taking it as an antioxidant on your own initiative; larger doses and injections of vitamin C may be prescribed by your doctor.

Side effects: Doses higher than 500 mg have been associated with diarrhea, rebound deficiency, and cancer promotion.

Caveats: Use high doses of vitamin C with care. Megadoses are popular, but some recent reports have implicated higher doses with *increased* cancer risks.

Vitamin D

Vitamin D builds and maintains teeth and bones; your body can't use calcium without D. A deficiency causes rickets in children and *osteomalacia* (bone softening) and *osteoporosis* (bone thinning) in adults. Studies suggest that vitamin D may fit into and inactivate certain cancer-promoting cells, blocking cancer tumor growth.

Canned salmon, egg yolks, greens, organ meats, and fish are all good sources. Be sure to spend fifteen minutes a day in the sun as well, because vitamin-D metabolism is dependent upon sunlight. Unfortunately, many Americans do not get enough sunlight to make D. Many people use sunscreen habitually, and this filters out the necessary UV rays. The dark skins of many African Americans also screen out much of the D-producing light, so they must be careful to get extra vitamin D from foods or supplements. Americans who live at latitudes above 40 degrees (imagine a belt extending from Boston through New York and Oregon) cannot make vitamin D during the winter. The essential UV component of light is scattered at too oblique an angle for our bodies to use. Finally, our bodies produce the vitamin less efficiently as we age, so getting enough from food is especially important if you are over fifty or live in northern climates. Cirrhosis also causes a deficiency.

VITAMIN D SUPPLEMENT

What it does: Vitamin D maintains liver health, discouraging the progression of hepatitis to cirrhosis.

How it works: Vitamin D bolsters the immune system, thereby lessening liver-tissue damage.

Who this should benefit: People older than 50, African Americans, and people who live in cold climates during the winter months.

Who should avoid this: No known groups.

Recommended formulation: Capsules.

Usual dosage range: 400 to 800 IU a day. More than 1,000 IU may be toxic.

Side effects: Overdoses cause excess calcium in the body, bone weakening, suppression of the immune system, and heart palpitations. Very high doses of D can impair immune response.

Caveats: Be sure to get fifteen minutes of sunlight daily— *without* sunscreen. If you use antibiotic ointments containing vitamin D, reduce your vitamin-D supplementation.

Vitamin E

Vitamin E (dl-alpha-tocopherol) helps build red blood cells and muscles. Several studies strongly suggest that this antioxidant vitamin helps prevent cancer and heart disease as well. Vitamin E bolsters the white blood cells of the immune system. In addition, the *Journal of the American Medical Association* has reported that vitamin E discourages liver fibrosis in older people. Vitamin E is found in cooked green leafy vegetables, poultry, seafood, wheat germ, oatmeal, vegetable oils (safflower, soybean oils), and nuts.

VITAMIN E SUPPLEMENT

What it does: Vitamin E plays major roles in cancer prevention and treatment. It slows cirrhosis and helps prevent cancerous liver changes.

How it works: By exerting powerful effects against free radicals, this fat-soluble antioxidant vitamin discourages cancerous changes and tissue damage. In addition, vitamin E enhances the activity of white blood cells and resistance to diseases, including cancer.

Who this should benefit: Vitamin E helps people with hepatitis C by slowing the progression of liver damage and cancer. E may help people undergoing chemotherapy for liver cancer by eliminating digestive-tract ulcers.

Who should avoid this: Not known.

Recommended formulation: The natural capsules (dL-alpha-tocopherol) contain more active ingredient than the manufactured variety.

Usual dosage range: 600 to 1,200 IU daily.

Side effects: Blood pressure increases.

Caveats: People with hypertension should not take vitamin E supplements unless their physicians advise it.

TPGS (tocopherol polyethylene glycol supplement), a special water-soluble form of vitamin E

What it does: TPGS helps deliver the fat-soluble vitamin E to people who can't absorb it from food or from conventional supplements; TPGS also enables the person with cirrhosis to absorb and use vitamins A, D, E, and K.

How it works: TPGS contains a form of vitamin E that enables the bodies of people with liver disease to absorb fat-soluble vitamins in an easily absorbed liquid form.

Who this should benefit: The one in five people with advanced hepatitis C who are deficient in vitamins A, D, and E. Their livers often make too little bile to process fat-soluble vitamins, so taking regular supplement capsules will not correct the deficiency. People undergoing chemotherapy for liver cancer also should benefit.

Who should avoid this: People whose livers can process fat-soluble vitamins.

Recommended formulation: Liquid; as the liver recovers, it may be possible to switch back to fat-soluble forms of the vitamins.

Usual dosage range: Varies, depending upon individual bile production.

Side effects: No serious effects at therapeutic levels. Overdose can cause bone pain, bone loss, nausea, vomiting, weakness, and calcium deposits on the heart and kidneys.

Caveats: Vitamins A and D are quite toxic, so it is important to take TPGS only as directed.

Vitamin K

Vitamin K promotes blood clotting and bone growth. Intestinal bacteria manufacture it, and we can derive it from green leafy vegetables and whole grains such as wheat bran and oats. Cabbage and organ meats are also good sources. A vitamin-K-deficient diet leads to liver damage, so clearly K is an important vitamin for someone with hepatitis C.

VITAMIN K SUPPLEMENT

What it does: Vitamin K is necessary for proper blood clotting.

How it works: The liver uses vitamin K to make the prothrombin necessary for blood clotting.

Who this should benefit: Anyone with hepatitis C, especially people with esophageal varices, which bleed easily.

Who should avoid this: No groups identified.

Recommended formulation: Capsule, liquid, or intravenous injection.

Usual dosage range: Large amounts, up to five times the RDA.

Side effects: No serious effects at therapeutic levels.

Caveats: Adding vitamin K to the diet of a person with liver damage may not always remedy a deficiency, because the problem is not a lack of K but the injured liver's inability to metabolize it.

MINERALS

Several minerals are important in the liver-friendly diet. Some, such as selenium and potassium, support your liver during therapy or delay the progression of tissue damage. Others, such as iron, may worsen your condition. Below you will find details of mineral supplements that are important in the management of hepatitis C.

Potassium and Salt

People without cirrhosis can safely eat the 3,000 milligrams, or about one teaspoonful, of salt recommended by the NAS. **If severe cirrhosis develops,** you will have to restrict your salt intake further. Salt impairs a damaged liver's ability to regulate fluid, so that the liver sends aberrant hormone messages that sabotage your body's precise salt-water balance. The liver tells the body to conserve water and salt. But salt soaks up water like a sponge, retaining fluid in the abdomen (ascites) and chest and ankles (edema).

To get rid of this extra fluid, you must flush water and restrict salt. Diuretics such as Aldactone, Lasix, and Midamore cause your body to excrete salt and water. Too much salt will counteract the effect of the diuretic, so your doctor will probably restrict you to ingesting only 2,000 to 2,500 milligrams of salt—less than a teaspoonful a day. Some people have to curtail their fluid intake, too.

Salt and potassium levels must remain balanced. Too little potassium can lead to a heart attack, so your doctor may prescribe potassium supplements or administer special diuretic combinations to maintain potassium as your body expels excess water and salt.

POTASSIUM CHLORIDE; also, POTASSIUM

What it does: Helps dispel ascites (abdominal swelling) and edema (leg swelling).

How it works: Potassium chloride, or KCl, is used like table salt to season food. The sodium found in salt retains water like a sponge, but in KCl, potassium replaces it. This switch helps you to expel excess bodily fluids by limiting sodium without losing potassium.

Who this should benefit: People with ascites and edema.

Who should avoid this: Use potassium or KCl only if your doctor, nutritionist, or dietitian recommends it; otherwise it could cause or exacerbate heart problems.

Recommended formulation: KCl consists of small crystals that look, taste, and are used like salt.

Usual dosage range: Use KCl like salt—up to 2,500 mg daily.

Side effects: Potassium affects heart function: Overdose can lead to serious heart problems, including heart attack.

Caveats: Don't use KCl if you have kidney problems (common in people with hepatitis C). Don't use KCl if your doctor has prescribed potassium-only supplements or potassium-sparing diuretics, such as Midamore and Aldactone. Some people dislike the taste of KCl.

Selenium

Selenium enhances immunity and resistance to cancer. A meta-analysis of twenty-seven countries found that people who take in the highest amounts of selenium have the lowest numbers of cancers. Selenium is found in organ meats, garlic, whole-grain breads, cereals, and legumes.

SELENIUM SUPPLEMENT

What it does: Discourages the progression of liver damage.

How it works: Enhances immunity and bolsters the body's immune defenses against cancer.

Who this should benefit: People with little liver damage: Selenium discourages cirrhosis and cancer formation in people with HCV.

Who should avoid this: Not known.

Recommended formulation: Your doctor or nutritional advisor may recommend an inorganic form, such as sodium selenite, if you are at high cancer risk. Otherwise, he or she may recommend the organic form of selenium, which is less toxic.

Usual dosage range: 250 mcg daily.

Side effects: Higher doses can produce fatigue, headache, dizziness, and a garlicky smell to the breath and urine.

Caveats: Some news reports have touted huge doses of selenium to prevent cancer, but the mineral can be toxic in doses higher than 300 mcg.

Iron

Don't take an iron supplement unless your doctor says it is necessary. High blood-iron levels have been linked to a greater likelihood of developing cirrhosis or cancer. Here's why: Just as our bodies need iron to function, the HCV virus requires iron to reproduce itself. When you have an infection, your blood-iron level dips—a smart move on your body's part to withhold the metal from the invading organism. Fifteen years ago, Tufts University scientists observed that hepatitis B and hepatitis C patients who had higher blood-iron levels were more likely to develop a chronic infection than those with lower levels. Other research has established that people with a large supply of iron in their livers are also the people who develop liver fibrosis, cirrhosis, and cancer. The National Health and Nutrition Examination Survey (NHANES) established that high iron levels are associated with higher cancer risks. Nine different studies involving 434 people with HCV found that those with a large supply of iron in their livers were less likely to respond to interferon therapy. On the other hand, those with no detectable iron were most likely to have the best outcome.

African Americans are more likely to have high iron levels than other ethnic groups, and this iron overload may be partly responsible for their poorer prognosis compared to other ethnic groups. People with a genetic condition called *hemochromatosis,* characterized by high iron levels, also tend to fare poorly with HCV.

Iron may wreak its havoc by encouraging oxidative damage that uses up protective antioxidants. It may also impair immunity directly by hobbling T-lymphocyte cells. But until a large, well-designed clinical trial is performed, we won't know for sure whether or how it sabotages liver health.

Meanwhile, there are steps you can take to protect yourself.

A simple blood test will tell your physician whether you have high iron levels. Everyone diagnosed with hepatitis C should ask for this test, and if you are African American, you *must* have your blood-iron level tested.

If your levels are high, your doctor can reduce them by *chelation,* a chemical process in which substances are introduced into the body that "escort" the iron out, lowering your blood-iron levels. A chelation study demonstrated that reducing the iron levels in the body of people with chronic hepatitis C lowered ALT levels dramatically by itself, without any other type of therapy.

Calcium

CALCIUM SUPPLEMENT

What it does: Protects against bone thinning and bone softening in people with cirrhosis and liver cancer, who are often
calcium-deficient.

How it works: Calcium works with vitamin D to prevent bone
cell loss.

Who this should benefit: People whose nausea makes it
impossible to get sufficient calcium from foods; also, people
who are vitamin-D deficient, especially the elderly and African
Americans.

Who should avoid this: No problems identified.

Recommended formulation: A variety of capsules, pills, and
liquids. The liquid formulations include calcium citrate and some
antacids, which also supply calcium for people with nausea.
Most calcium supplements also have 100 to 200 IU vitamin D,
because your body cannot absorb calcium if you are vitamin-D-
deficient.

Usual dosage range: Premenopausal women need at least 800
mg daily, and postmenopausal women who are not on estrogen
therapy need 1,200 mg. Check the label for the amount of
"bioavailable calcium."

Side effects: Overdose causes constipation and toxicity.

Caveats: Choose refined or chelated calcium and avoid
supplements from dolomite, which are sometimes adulterated
with lead, a toxic metal.

Magnesium

MAGNESIUM SUPPLEMENT

What it does: Remedies muscle weakness, fatigue, nausea,
and vomiting when due to magnesium deficiency.

How it works: Restores this essential mineral, which is often
depleted in people with liver disease.

Who this should benefit: People who have low magnesium
because of a poor diet, nausea, vomiting, or the use of diuretics.

Who should avoid this: No problems identified.

Recommended formulation: Magnesium gluconate liquid.

Usual dosage range: 500 mg 3 times a day.

Side effects: Too much magnesium can cause heart attacks.

Caveats: If you take a magnesium supplement, don't take laxatives: many contain magnesium and can contribute to an overdose.

Zinc

Zinc may improve immunity and foster cancer resistance. In people with HCV, too little zinc may cause encephalopathy. Zinc deficiencies go hand-in-hand with lowered immunity, but so does an overdose. Zinc overdose also seems to encourage bacterial infection and certain cancers. Be careful with zinc supplements, because you need to preserve a delicate balance between selenium and zinc. Unless *specific* conditions dictate otherwise, take no more than 15 milligrams of zinc daily, which you can easily derive from food in the form of wheat germ, oatmeal, nuts, oysters, clams, spinach, mushrooms, and liver.

ZINC SUPPLEMENT

What it does: Stimulates the appetite and supports immune defenses.

How it works: Zinc supplements help maintain weight because zinc restores the senses of smell and taste when these have been lost to zinc deficiency. It also boosts the activity of killer cells and lymphocytes, two important immune-system components.

Who this should benefit: People who have lost their senses of taste and smell; also, people whose hair quality has suffered as a side effect of interferon.

Recommended formulation: Zinc sulfate, zinc acetate tablets or capsules.

Usual dosage range: 15 to 100 mg a day, sometimes as much as 600 mg a day.

Time span of therapy: For no more than one month.

Caveats: Using zinc for more than a month depletes the body's copper stores and may encourage bacterial infections.

Side effects: Nausea, diarrhea.

PROTEIN SUPPLEMENTS

PROTEIN SUPPLEMENT DRINKS. These drinks contain special protein building blocks called branched-chain amino acids, such as isoleucine, leucine, and valine.

What they do: Several studies have shown that a protein supplement drink with a high proportion of branched-chain amino acids reduces the incidence of encephalopathy. It may also reduce infection.

How they work: Branched-chain amino acids are less likely to lower the levels of ammonia, a toxic by-product of protein metabolism. Ammonia causes encephalopathy by distorting the brain's neurotransmitters, or chemical messengers.

Who this should benefit: Anyone at risk for encephalopathy, such as people with hepatitis-C-induced liver damage.

Who should avoid this: Not known.

Recommended formulation: Varies, but usually a liquid that includes branched-chain amino acids, sugar, and special fats.

Usual dosage range: Varies with size and liver condition.

Side effects: None.

Caveats: The drugs *lactulose* and *neomycin* also lower ammonia levels and are often given along with these supplements.

Fat Supplements

I was steadily losing weight and couldn't seem to eat enough to gain it back. I was beginning to look gaunt, though I'm only 33! I'm convinced that MCT oil saved my life. I cook with it, put it in my food, and it allows me to eat more heartily without feeling sick. I've maintained a weight that looks just right and I look better than ever before.

Alanna

MCT OIL SUPPLEMENT

What it is: MCT is an acronym for *medium-chain triglyc-erides,* fat building blocks that are specially structured for easy absorption by those who produce too little bile. MCT oil formulations usually add *structured lipids,* nutritionally complete oils that can enhance immunity.

What it does: Provides easily digested fats, enhances the immune system, inhibits tumor cell growth in the laboratory, and discourages artery disease.

How it works: MCT oil does not require bile for absorption into the bloodstream, so it doesn't cause nausea in people who are usually nauseated by fats.

Who this should benefit: People with cirrhosis or liver damage.

Who should avoid this: Diabetics, people with profound malnutrition, and people who are taking blood thinners.

Recommended formulation: Capsules; also found in nutritional drink supplements such as MaxEPA, MegaEPA, and Promega. MCT oil can also can be used in cooking.

Usual dosage range: 3 to 6 180-mg capsules daily; as recommended for cooking.

Side effects: Using MCT alone can produce diarrhea and heartburn. MCT oil can disrupt blood-sugar levels in diabetics.

Caveats: MCT oil can interfere with blood clotting, so get your doctor's prior approval if you are taking blood-thinning medications such as Coumadin (warfarin) or if you are a diabetic. If MCT is the only fat in your diet, you should also take the essential fatty acid *linoleic acid*.

High-Calorie Supplements

Suplena and other high-calorie supplement drinks; other brand names include **Ensure, Ultra Slim Fast, Sweet Success,** and **Boost**.

What they do: Prevent malnutrition in people who cannot eat normal portions of food or who cannot eat solid food without nausea.

How they work: A large glassful of liquid is infused with calories, fats, protein, minerals, and fiber.

Who this should benefit: People made nauseous by interferon therapy, cirrhosis, or other liver damage.

Who should avoid this: Use these supplements only if your doctor, dietitian, or nutritionist recommends them.

Recommended formulation: Liquid.

Usual dosage range: Varies; usually 1 to 2 cans a day.

Side effects: These drinks are only a temporary answer to malnutrition. They don't contain enough fiber, nor do they provide every trace nutrient and phytochemical that is necessary to good health.

Caveats: Most high-calorie drinks are rich in vitamins and minerals, so don't drink them regularly without your doctor's or dietitian's knowledge. The vitamins and minerals you are taking, added to those in the drink, could create overdoses of some nutrients and "rebound" deficiencies of others.

Other Dietary Supplements

Colostrum is the nutritious milklike fluid produced by a mother in the three to four days immediately after childbirth. It is high in antibodies, lactoferrin, lymphocytes, and macrophages, and studies suggest that it transfers important immunities to breast-fed infants. Kenneth Singleton, M.D., MPH, uses colostrum from cows to support immune function in the livers of people with hepatitis C. Be sure to buy colostrum derived from cows raised without antibiotics, such as Symbiotics New Life Colostrum. The usual dose is 1 teaspoonful of powder or one tablet twice a day. **Grape seed extract,** or **Pycnogenol,** is a powerful antioxidant that protects the liver from cirrhosis and liver cancer. The supplement pycnogenol with a small "p" is often extracted from grape seeds and contains antioxidants called polyphenols, flavonoids, or proanthocyanidins. Pycnogenol with a capital "P" is a specific mixture of natural antioxidant flavonoids obtained from the pine tree *Pinus pinaster*.

Supplements to Avoid

If you have hepatitis C, avoid **vitamin A** supplements in favor of beta-carotene: Vitamin A causes liver toxicity, and, as noted on page 129, you cannot overdose from beta-carotene, as you may from vitamin A. Avoid **niacin,** vitamin B_3, because as described on page 130, it can encourage liver damage. Too much **manganese** may cause encephalopathy and has been implicated in the development of Parkinson's disease. Your dietary counselor may change your diet or supplementation regimen to minimize manganese exposure. **Omega-3 fatty acids** are packaged in supplements labeled "Omega-3," "EPA and DHA," or "Linolenic Acid." If you cannot tolerate fatty fish, then omega-3 oil supplements may benefit you. But you should take your omega-3 oils from food if you can. Studies have shown that although people who ate omega-3-rich foods such as salmon and mackerel enjoyed significant health benefits, people who took an equivalent amount in supplements did not. Also, people who take omega-3 oil in addition to their regular diets are adding unwanted fat to their diets.

Nondietary Supplements

SAM-e (S-adenosyl-methionine). SAM-e plays many roles in the functioning of a healthy liver. If SAM-e is depleted, the liver cannot make bile or needed amino acids, nor can it rid itself of methionine, which builds up to toxic levels. SAM-e regulates fat and fluid content, preventing fat deposits from settling on the liver in a condition called fatty liver, which was described in Chapter 1. In fact, SAM-e is the first supplement shown to reverse the dangerous deposition of fat on the liver. In 1990, the team of S. Rafique at the Royal Free Hospital School of Medicine London followed 24 patients with chronic liver disease. The number of cholesterol deposits on the livers of 10 of the SAM-e patients fell, but only 4 of the placebo group had fewer cholesterol deposits. A 1992 Japanese study by H. Kakimoto of 16 patients given 600 milligrams of SAM-e IV for two weeks found that SAM-e improved the ability of liver cell membranes to transport needed fluids and substances: This is often compromised by cirrhosis in people with hepatitis C. A 1990 study of 1,000 patients published in the *Postgraduate Medical Journal* suggests that giving SAM-e both orally and via IV increases its benefits without side effects. The usual dose ranges from 200 to 800 milligrams once daily.

Alpha-lipoic acid is an antioxidant that helps to support liver metabolism and discourages cancer formation. It also helps the liver to purge dangerously high amounts of heavy metals such as iron, copper, lead, and mercury from the body. Stores of lipoic acid drop as you age, so middle-aged persons with hepatitis C probably need lipoic acid supplements.

MSM (methyl sulfonyl methane) bolsters the liver's health by fortifying the immune system. Levels of MSM drop as one ages, so supplements are important for older people with hepatitis C. MSM also fortifies collagen and connective tissue, which can become degraded in people with cirrhosis.

Accessory nutrients help B-complex vitamins transform food energy into forms that cells can use. **Choline, inositol,** and **coenzyme Q-10** (also called Q10 and ubiquinone) are other B-complex accessories that are closely related to B vitamins. Coenzyme Q-10 prevents the liver cells' mitochondria, the cells' energy factories, from damage by free radicals. Most studies of coenzyme Q-10 center on its role in preventing heart disease. Heart patients who are given coenzyme Q-10 recover from surgery with fewer complications; this finding may be germane to people with hepatitis C who face surgery for liver cancer or who face transplantation surgery. **PABA (para-aminobenzoic acid)** and **substance P** work similarly with vitamin C to prevent cancer.

Transfer factor, a substance made from the leukocytes, or white blood cells, is so named because it "transfers" an allergic reaction from one person to another. Transfer factor treats long-term infections such as hepatitis C as well as some immune-system diseases. Transfer factor also discourages tumor growth in patients with liver cancer.

UltraClear and **UltraClear Plus** are compounds that have been patented by HealthComm to detoxify the liver. Dr. Single-ton uses UltraClear to enhance the liver's ability to detoxify drugs and foreign substances. UltraClear helps people with chronic hepatitis C to minimize drug side effects and reduce environmental poisoning from liver-toxic chemicals.

For more information

Bibliography

Bland, Jeffrey, Ph.D. *Choline, Lecithin, Inositol, and Other "Accessory" Nutrients*. Keats Publishing, 1982.

Goldberg, Burton. *Alternative Medicine: The Definitive Guide*. Future Medicine Publishing, 1993.

Katzenstein, Larry. *Secrets of St. John's Wort*. Hodder & Stoughton, 1998.

Lee, William H., R.Ph., Ph.D. *Co-enzyme Q-10*. Keats Publishing, 1987.

Mitchell, Deborah. *The SAM-e Solution: The Essential Guide to the Revolutionary Antidepression Supplement*. Warner Books, 1999.

Passwater, Richard, Ph.D. *Lipoic Acid: The Metabolic Antioxidant*. Keats Publishing, 1995.

Wright, J., M.D., *Dr. Wright's Guide to Healing with Nutrition*. Keats Publishing, 1990.

Organizations

United States Department of Agriculture
14 Independence Avenue, SW
Washington, DC 20250
(202) 606-8000
Web site: www.usda.gov
Provides nutrient information.

CHAPTER SEVEN

Herbs

Many people who are discouraged by interferon's low long-term effectiveness or profound side effects may wonder, "Are herbal remedies good medicine for liver problems such as hepatitis C?" The answer is yes—but you must be careful. As you will see, you can find healing at the herbalist's, but you must take herbs with the same care you use for conventional medications. This chapter will help you to safely explore effective herbal remedies, even if you are simultaneously undergoing interferon therapy. Although in its most narrow definition, an herb is a soft-stemmed shrub, this chapter refers to any plant used for healing purposes.

A copious amount of high-quality research demonstrates that herbs can help improve liver health, but none has yet shown that any herbal remedy can cure hepatitis C. Cure, however, is not the only goal of herbal treatment. There is compelling evidence that herbs such as milk thistle can boost the immune system, discourage liver injury, and slow the progression to cirrhosis. All this may make you feel better and may delay or prevent complications such as cirrhosis and liver cancer. In Chapter 9, "Putting It All Together," you will read examples of how specific herbs have helped people with hepatitis C to sustain or to regain their health.

But even if an herb simply helps you feel well enough to complete interferon therapy, isn't that in itself a worthwhile goal?

If you followed the suggestions in Chapter 4 for finding a physician who is open to alternative therapies, he or she can help you decide which herbs are right for you. This is important, because some scientists and clinicians sneer at all herbal treatments. They are, however, ignoring important facts.

First, fully 25 percent of the medications approved by the Food and Drug Administration (FDA), as listed in the 1999 *United States Pharmacopoeia,* are extracted from plants or are copies of plant chemicals, or *phytochemicals.* Often we learned of them from native peoples who used plants as their drugstore. Many of these drugs are as familiar as aspirin, derived from white willow bark and meadowsweet. We have also distilled morphine from poppies, the birth control pill from Mexican yams, the anticancer medication vincristine from periwinkle, and taxol from the Pacific yew. Our own pharmacies offer evidence that herbs can treat and heal when they are properly selected and safely applied.

Secondly, many clinicians say that there is not enough scientific evidence for the effectiveness of herbs and point to a dearth of in-depth studies. They point out that herbalists often rely upon anecdotes about patients who have been "cured" by herbs, buttressed by biochemical theories about how the plants work. Without large numbers of carefully selected patients in controlled and duplicated studies, they say, we don't know whether to credit the treatment or some coincident factor.

It is true that we need to test herbs the same way we test FDA-approved medications, with double-blind controlled studies. But it is also true that in this country the task—and large cost—of organizing and underwriting such studies falls largely to pharmaceutical companies. Because herbal medications cannot be patented, private companies are rarely interested in sponsoring a lengthy, expensive research and development program for an herb that cannot be profited from. Such companies, which spend

$231 million annually on drug development, fear they will not be able to recoup their expenses.

But this research vacuum may be filled soon, because herbal treatments are becoming more popular. In 1995, Americans spent $4 billion on botanical products, and that rate has increased by as much as 100 percent annually. This sizable investment has piqued the interest of drug companies, and a few have ventured into the herbal market to fund such testing, research, and development. More companies will soon follow suit. In the meantime, it is up to the government to test some common herbs.

This has already begun, slowly in our country and very extensively in Germany, whose Commission E, a division of the Bundesgesundheitsamt (state medical agency), has published more than three hundred monographs evaluating hundreds of herbal treatments by exacting Western scientific standards. Rigorous Western-style research elsewhere has already found that herbs can help common conditions that conventional medicines cannot treat. For example, a 1998 Australian study found that Chinese herbal treatments are effective against irritable-bowel syndrome, a gastrointestinal disorder that is common in industrialized countries and for which conventional medicine offers only symptomatic relief. A similar study found that saw palmetto eases men's symptoms of prostate enlargement.

How to Use Herbs Safely

Effectiveness is just one key issue in evaluating medicinal herbs; safety is another. There are safety issues to consider with herbs, just as there are with conventional medications.

It's easy to take herbs safely. Many prominent alternative-medicine spokespersons say that herbs are milder and safer than conventional medications. This generalization is usually true as long as you take the herb correctly, as your herbal practitioner and doctor recommend. The key is to follow expert advice, take only the recommended dosage, and consult with your doctor to avoid drug interactions.

The FDA tests new conventional medications vigorously before it allows them on your pharmacist's shelf, but it issues warnings about herbal medicines only after someone has been harmed. All this means that you must be at least as careful about herbs as you are about conventional medications. If you take too much or take an herb without expert approval, you can risk poisoning, drug interactions, or serious side effects.

Here are some tips for taking herbs safely:

1. **Involve your doctor.** Hepatitis C is a serious chronic disease, and although many herbs can protect your liver and improve its functioning, an herb can sometimes mask signs that your liver is worsening. A 1997 survey reported in the *Journal of the American Medical Association* revealed that 15 million Americans take herbs at the same time they are taking prescription medicines. Sixty percent don't tell their doctor, so he or she can't monitor them for interactions.

   Your first stop should be your doctor, who should be able to advise you himself or herself or refer you appropriately: Half of the doctors in America now practice some form of alternative medicine and will refer you to alternative practitioners such as herbalists. Because an herb may interact with interferon or affect your lab test values, you need the same team approach you adopt with conventional medicine.

   Also, the enzyme levels of people with hepatitis C sometimes go up and down with or without treatment, and this fluctuation may lead people to believe that an herb is helping them when their disease would be waxing and waning anyway. Your doctor can examine you to tell whether an herb is helping or whether it is time to try another.

   The information in this chapter is no substitute for the care of a licensed physician. The only way to know whether an herbal treatment is working for you is to obtain regular medical care and testing from a licensed physician and to carefully follow your doctor's advice.

2. **Choose an herbal professional.** Don't take herbal recommendations from anyone but an herbalist with credentials

and years of training, just as you would demand in a physician. For tips on finding the best practitioners, first look for a member of the American Herbalists Guild (their address is given at the end of this chapter). Despite the exhortation of herbal books, herbalism for hepatitis C is not a do-it-yourself project. Western herbalists tend to use *simples,* individual herbs that address specific problems, such as cirrhosis. Many people with HCV find that individual liver-friendly herbs described herein support the effectiveness of or help reduce the side effects of interferon.

But those herbalists trained in Oriental medicine tend to use several herbs blended carefully in concert, which is impossible for the uninitiated to do safely. (See "Other Herbal Systems," below.) The herbal combination changes in a complicated manner as the patient progresses, and the combined action of herbs is quite complex; sometimes small amounts of normally toxic herbs are even added to the mix. This is definitely a strategy for experienced professionals only.

OTHER HERBAL SYSTEMS

This chapter describes the use of herbs based upon modern Western concepts and traditions. But every people, from the ancient Egyptians and Icelanders to the North American Indians who preceded us, has developed their own system of herbal medicine. Two systems, Ayurvedic herbal medicine and traditional Chinese medicine (TCM), are in common practice in the West.

Ayurvedic Herbal Medicine
According to this ancient Indian medical theory, there are five elements—fire, water, earth, air, and ether. Each has a counterpart in the elements that define the health of the human body. These bodily elements join to produce the three *doshas,* or three humors. *Vata* represents air or movement or wind; *pitta* is fire, for example, bile production by the liver; and *kapha* is water, for

example, phlegm. Healing is achieved by balancing the three doshas.

The taste of an herb—sweet, sour, salty, pungent, bitter, or astringent—determines its healing properties. An astringent herb, for example, is thought to cool pitta, or fire, and would be helpful in treating liver inflammations, such as that caused by hepatitis C.

Traditional Chinese Medicine (TCM)

TCM also incorporates five elements and is also based upon taste. The five elements of this system are fire, earth, metal, water, and wood, each with its own complement in the body. The taste of an herb determines its action on the body. A "fire" herb tastes bitter, a "water" herb is salty, "wood" is sour, and so on. Herbs without a pronounced taste are categorized as "bland" and are often thought to be effective in ridding the body of excess water, which becomes important in treating the ascites and edema that afflict many people with liver damage from hepatitis C. Temperature is another indicator of herb action; TCM divides medicinal plants into hot, warm, neutral, cool, and cold herbs.

As in Ayurvedic herbalism, the aim of TCM is to achieve health through achieving balance. To this end, the concept of two complementary energies, *yin* and *yang,* is ascribed to many foods and herbs. Complex herbal mixtures are prescribed by TCM practitioners in an attempt to restore balance of elements, tastes, temperature, and yin and yang.

3. **Choose standardized formulations of herbs.** These allow you to be sure that you are receiving the correct dose of the herb each time you take it.

    Plucking or growing your own herbs is tricky because the amount and proportion of active ingredients varies according to soil, weather, and genetics. You could also end up with a "look-alike" herb that has unwanted biochemical actions. Instead, your doctor or herbalist will guide you to a reliable source.

HERBAL FORMULATIONS

Decoctions: The hardiest parts of the herb, including roots and bark, are boiled in water for ten minutes, then allowed to steep.

Infusions: Boiling water is poured over the petals, flowers, or leaves of an herb; the mixture is allowed to steep for at least twenty minutes, then strained.

Tinctures: Alcohol is used to extract the medicinal properties of an herb. Dried or fresh herbs are mixed with alcohol, and this preparation stands for two to six weeks.

Extracts: Extracts are prepared like tinctures, except that water is used as the extraction medium.

Capsules: You can buy a concentration of most herbs in capsule form.

---

4. **Look for GRAS, the FDA's green light.** The FDA has partially evaluated many herbs and has placed 250 on its "generally recognized as safe," or GRAS, list.
5. **Be especially careful when giving herbs to children.** Always get your pediatrician's approval before giving your child herbs, even in smaller amounts. Children often metabolize chemicals differently than adults, whether the chemicals are natural or pharmaceutical. An herb that does not harm an adult's liver might injure a child. Check with your obstetrician before using herbs if you are pregnant, because few rigorous scientific tests have been conducted on their safety for unborn children.

   If you are nursing, you can find the most accurate, comprehensive, and up-to-date treatment of the effects of herbs on breast milk in *Breastfeeding,* by Ruth A. Lawrence,

M.D., and Robert M. Lawrence, M.D. (Mosby, 1999). The chief known effects on breast milk are noted within the discussions of individual liver herbs below.

6. **Be an online skeptic.** Many Internet sites are rife with medical misinformation; herbal and alternative-therapy sites are no exception. Discuss any intriguing online discoveries with your physician.

HERBS THAT TREAT HEPATITIS

Hepatitis C is too new a diagnosis to have a long herbal history, but herbs have been successfully used to treat hepatitis, cirrhosis, and related liver ailments through many years and many lands. Chief among them are milk thistle, licorice, yarrow, and skullcap. But you should also know about other herbs that can seriously damage the liver, so some are described on page 167. As you read through this guide, pay careful attention to recommended dosages and side effects.

MILK THISTLE, or ST. MARY'S THISTLE
Botanical name: Silybum marianum.

What it is: A liver-protective herb in the daisy family, milk thistle is often considered a nuisance weed, but is golden to hepatitis C sufferers. It exudes a milky juice.

What it does: Extensive German research offers copious evidence that milk thistle, particularly its seeds, protects the liver from toxins. Milk thistle contains a variety of *flavonlignand* compounds, notably *silybinin, silychristin,* and *silydianin,* which are collectively called *silymarin*. Early German animal and *in vitro* studies showed liver regeneration in rats and petri dishes. The herb's active ingredient, silybinin, protected the livers of rats given the poisonous "Death Cap" mushroom (*Amanita phalloides*), which destroys the livers of and kills 40 percent of its victims even after prompt medical care. Milk thistle prevented liver destruction even when given hours after ingestion, when liver damage had begun. In hundreds of studies since 1969, including more than fifty double-blind human studies involving thousands of patients, milk thistle has been shown to protect and repair the liver against a wide variety of liver damage, from mushroom poisoning to chemical damage. When 170 people with cirrhosis were given silymarin in 1991, they proved more likely to survive than those who received a placebo. A Finnish hospital study found that when 170 people with liver damage were given silymarin, their liver enzymes fell more than the liver enzymes of 50 control patients who were not given the herb. But we don't know whether the liver enzyme tests necessarily mean the underlying disease is being treated.

The U.S. government is now investigating milk thistle to determine whether it reduces liver damage.

How it works: Silymarin compounds bind to liver cell membranes and act as antioxidants against free-radical damage and damage from internal and external toxins. Milk-thistle seeds contain betaine, which may also protect the liver, and fatty acids that may reduce inflammation.

Milk thistle is thought to protect the liver by (1) changing the exterior membrane of liver cells so that liver poisons can't enter and (2) stimulating the liver cells to manufacture more protein. This dual action serves to accelerate the natural regenerating capacity if the liver and liver cells produce the enzymes the liver needs to recover function. Milk thistle may help those on interferon therapy.

Who should benefit: People with both acute and chronic hepatitis as well as people with chemical injury such as overexposure to dry-cleaning fluids.

Who should avoid this: Pregnant and nursing mothers should seek their doctors' approval.

Recommended formulation: Standardized extract.

Usual dosage range: 1 to 2 tablets daily of the standardized extract of 80 percent silymarin and 20 percent water; 100 mg 2 to 3 times daily of the standardized extract containing 10 percent silymarin, 90 percent water; or 1 dropperful 2 to 3 times daily of the nonstandardized liquid extract. Silymarin is not naturally water-soluble, so avoid teas, which are too weak for effectiveness.

Time span of therapy: Results appear in 1 to 3 months.

Side effects: Mild laxative effect, headache.

Caveats: Most studies lump together people with a variety of liver diseases, so more-focused studies should be performed to see whether silymarin is especially effective against hepatitis C.

LICORICE

Botanical name: Glycyrrhiza glabra.

What it is: Real licorice isn't as common as we think. Unless it's imported, the black candy familiar to every child is likely to be flavored with anise instead. But we do encounter the real thing in laxatives and in "naturally sweetened" herb teas. Chinese physicians have used licorice for centuries to treat liver problems, including cirrhosis.

What it does: Licorice's active ingredient, *glycyrrhizinic acid,* promotes protective mucus. Like milk thistle, it protects the liver membrane and lowers blood ALT levels.

How it works: A recent study in *Microbiology and Immunology* indicated that glycyrrhizinic acid stimulates the liver cells' production of interferon. This, in turn, normalizes liver enzymes, resulting in a better prognosis for people with a hepatitis virus.

In Japan, the active ingredient is sold as SNMC—Stronger Neominophen C—an extract of licorice root. A 1997 cancer study by Yasuji Arase found SNMC effective in preventing hepatitis C from progressing to liver cancer. Over the 15-year course of the study, 25 percent of the high-risk patients developed liver cancer; only 12 percent of a comparable group treated with SNMC did.

Who this should benefit: People at risk for liver cirrhosis and cancer, including people with HCV.

Who should avoid this: Do not take when pregnant, if you are a diabetic, or if you have hypertension, glaucoma, heart disease, or stroke.

Recommended formulation: Powdered root; drug powder (glycyrrhizin); dry extracts for infusion.

Usual dosage range: The average daily dose is 5 to 15 g of the powdered root, or 200 to 600 mg of glycyrrhizin daily.

Time span of therapy: No longer than 6 weeks, to avoid pseudoaldosteronism, a serious condition that mimics steroid abuse.

Side effects: Licorice is on the FDA GRAS list. But too much licorice, more than 50 g a day, causes low potassium and high blood pressure, and has caused at least one case of cardiac arrest. Excessive doses, even from overindulging in real licorice candies, may also cause headache, lethargy, sodium and water retention, potassium loss, high or low blood pressure, and headache.

Caveats: Breastfeeding mothers should avoid excessive amounts of licorice.

Interferon alert: Licorice can stimulate your body to produce interferon. So if you are on interferon therapy, do not take licorice without discussing it with your physician, because you could end up with too large a cumulative dose.

ARTICHOKE, GLOBE ARTICHOKE

Botanical name: Cynara scolymus.

What it is: This edible plant so familiar to gourmets is, like milk thistle, a member of the daisy family. Its leaves and roots are used fresh or dried.

What it does: Artichokes contain *silymarin, cynaropicrin,* and *cynarin,* which may have anticancer activity, conceivably against liver cancer.

How it works: Western research shows cyanopicrin and cynarin protect the liver by stimulating bile production, which in turn lowers cholesterol and may discourage cancer. According to an August 1997 *Journal of the National Cancer Institute* report, when Case Western University researchers applied silymarin extract derived from artichoke to the skins of tumor-prone mice exposed to ultraviolet light, only 25 percent of the treated mice developed tumors. All the mice in the control group did.

Who should benefit: People with HCV; artichoke may slow liver damage and discourage cancer development.

Who should avoid this: Children and pregnant and lactating women.

Recommended formulation: Look for standardized dry extracts.

Usual dosage range: 6 g of the dried drug or 500 mg of the dry extract daily. Or take 1 tablespoonful of dried leaf in a cup of boiling water steeped for 10 minutes twice daily.

Time span of therapy: Varies, but your doctor will know whether it is working within a few months.

Side effects: None reported at properly applied therapeutic doses.

ASTRAGALUS GUMMIFER, also GUM DRAGON

Botanical name: Tragacanth.

What it is: The gum exudate from the tragacanth shrub, which grows in the Middle East. The dried gum forms flakes, which can be reconstituted in water to form a gelatin-like substance.

What it does: Retards liver damage and protects against liver cancer by increasing the activity of the immune system.

How it works: Astragalus contains saponins and half a dozen polysaccharides. These compounds pump up immune-system activity by several routes—they increase the number of *macrophages* (virus-eating white cells), and they increase the activity of macrophages. The polysaccharides also increase the number of *killer cells,* the immune-system components that actually kill viruses.

Who should benefit: People with both acute and chronic hepatitis C; astragalus has been especially effective as an adjunct treatment for people with extensive cirrhosis.

Who should avoid this: Pregnant and nursing mothers should seek their doctors' approval.

Recommended formulation: Standardized extract.

Usual dosage range: 1 or 2 tablets daily of the standardized extract, or 1 dropperful 2 times a day of the liquid extract.

Time span of therapy: Results appear in 1 to 3 months.

Side effects: Astragalus has a laxative effect.

Caveats: Allergic reactions occur but are very rare. Overdoses can be life-threatening.

GOLDEN SEAL

Botanical name: Hydrastis canadensis.

What it is: The dried rhizome and roots of this plant.

What it does: Native Americans introduced 19th-century pioneers to golden seal's antibiotic properties. They applied it to the skin as an antiseptic and used it internally for digestive problems.

How it works: Golden seal contains *berberine hydrastine,* which lowers inflammation of the mucous membranes. It also stimulates the flow of bile, which helps digest fats.

Who should benefit: People with symptoms of hepatitis, especially poor appetite, and people with gallstones.

Who should avoid this: Children; people with hypertension; heart, kidney, or spleen disease; diabetes or glaucoma; and people who have had a stroke. Golden seal may cause abortion.

Recommended formulation: 20 percent tincture of golden seal; powdered root.

Usual dosage range: ½ to 1 teaspoon of tincture or powdered root 2 to 3 times daily for no more than 10 days.

Time span of therapy: Two cycles of 10 days each separated by 10 days is the maximum course, unless your physician recommends more.

Side effects: This strong central-nervous-system stimulant can cause heart attacks or suppress breathing.

Caveats: Nursing mothers should not use golden seal. It has affected infants' blood pressure and caused irritation and nausea. Golden seal also disturbed the balance of the proteins albumin and bilirubin in nursing infants.

Like ginseng, golden seal is expensive, so adulteration with other plants is common. These contaminants often include bloodroot (*Sanguinaria canadensis*), which is also yellow and very toxic.

GINSENG. There are three biologically distinct types of "ginseng," each with a different botanical name.

Botanical names: Panax ginseng ("Asian," or "Korean," from

China, Korea, and Japan) and *Panax quinquefolius* (American ginseng) are very similar. They share the same genus, or botanical group, and are both widely used in China. *Eleutheroccus senticosus* (Siberian ginseng) is a member of another family and is not true ginseng, but has similar chemical constituents, so it is grouped with the true ginsengs. *E. senticosus* is used and studied less commonly than the true ginsengs in the East, but all three ginsengs are used interchangeably in the West.

What it is: Asian ginseng is cultivated in China, Korea, Japan, and Russia, where the mature roots (from a plant that is at least 6 years old) are prized as the "life root." American ginseng, grown in North America, is prized and widely used in China as well. Both have a plethora of uses and are considered "life extenders." Ginseng is also very expensive, at $200 a pound wholesale. Oriental medicine uses Siberian ginseng less extensively, often in herbal mixtures.

What it does: Asian and American ginseng protect the liver from alcohol, drugs, and other toxic substances. A Korean epidemiological study found lower rates of liver cancer in people who used ginseng powder, but not in users of fresh ginseng or of ginseng tea. Asian ginseng also improved liver function in a study of 24 elderly people suffering from cirrhosis.

How it works: The mechanism of *ginsenosides,* the chief active ingredients in every type of ginseng, is poorly understood, Ginsenosides are thought to stimulate the immune system by beefing up infection-fighting macrophages—white blood cells. They have antiviral activity as well. In human studies, they have eliminated herpes sores.

Who should benefit: American and Asian ginseng may help to protect people with hepatitis C from cirrhosis.

Who should avoid this: Pregnant or nursing women and women with fibrocystic (lumpy) breasts. Ginseng is an anticoagulant, so avoid it if you have a blood-clotting problem.

Recommended formulation: Use the Standard NF (the National Formulary) formulation for American and Asian ginseng, in comminuted drug powder, capsules, or tablets if you can find them. Many other formulations, such as nonstandardized powders, capsules, tablets, drug infusions, and teas, are available, but see "Caveat emptor" below.

Usual dosage range: ¼ to ½ teaspoonful of root powder twice a day. To make infusions of American and Asian ginseng, pour boiling water over 3 g of the comminuted drug, steep for 5 to 10 minutes, then strain and drink. The infusion may be taken 3 to 4 times a day.

The traditional Chinese medicine formula *Ginseng stomachic pills* (Ren Shen Jian Pi Wan) is often recommended for symptoms such as bloating, gas, irregular bowel movements, and the inability to gain weight. This formula contains citrus peel, ginseng atractylodes, barley spouts, and hawthorn. Six to ten small pills 3 times a day before meals are usually prescribed.

Time span of therapy: 3- to 4-week periods, separated by a 2-month period of abstinence. The length of the abstinent period may vary according to your doctor's or herbalist's advice.

Side effects: Ginseng is quite safe; in fact, it is on the FDA GRAS list. But don't use more than the recommended therapeutic dosages, because massive overdoses can bring on many side effects. Overdose can cause or worsen insomnia, allergy, hay fever, and asthma symptoms. Overdose also encourages high blood pressure and cardiac abnormalities.

Caveats: Nursing mothers should avoid ginseng because it is associated with transient sex-hormone imbalances in infants.

Caveat emptor: Buy ginseng from a source recommended by your herbalist or physician, because ginseng is an expensive herb, and adulteration is widespread. In a sampling of 54 U.S. health food stores, 60 percent of the samples contained too little ginseng to be effective, and 25 percent of the "ginseng" preparations contained no ginseng at all; many contained "desert ginseng," another, unrelated, herb. Asian or American ginseng must be harvested at full maturity—six years—and buying from a reliable source will increase your chance of obtaining an effective version of the herb.

DANDELION

Botanical name: Taraxacum officinale.

What it is: The roots and leaves of the familiar, hardy lawn weed. Dandelion has been a popular liver herb throughout Europe since the 15th century, but American Indians and 10th-century Arabians used it as well.

What it does: Like golden seal, dandelion promotes bile and fights infection.

How it works: Contains many biologically active compounds, including steroids and warfarin, a blood thinner.

Who this should benefit: Dandelion can be especially helpful to people with HCV who have kidney stones and gallstones (but only after seeing a physician to rule out certain complications). Dandelion also benefits people with appetite loss or intestinal distress, and people who are taking interferon.

Who should avoid this: People with biliary-duct problems, children, pregnant and nursing women.

Recommended formulation: Look for the tincture or extract for infusion.

Usual dosage range: 10 to 15 drops of the tincture up to 3 times daily. Begin at the lower dose. Or make an infusion with 1 tablespoon cut herb in 1 cup of boiling water. Steep 20 minutes.

Time span of therapy: 3 to 4 months.

Side effects: Dandelion is on the FDA GRAS list, but long-term use can cause potassium loss. It can also cause minor symptoms such as skin rash, diarrhea, and stomach upset.

Caveats: People with heart problems should use dandelion with care.

YARROW

Botanical name: Achillea millefolium.

What it is: Yarrow is a 3-foot perennial covered with delicate fuzzy hairs. Yarrow enjoys mythological fame as the plant Achilles used to stanch bleeding from a fellow warrior's wounds during the Trojan War. Achilles' Chinese contemporaries used all parts of the yarrow to combat inflammation and bleeding. In India, Ayurvedic healers used yarrow to lower fevers.

What it does: Two animal studies showed that yarrow protects the liver from toxic chemical damage. And a scientifically conducted human trial in India showed yarrow helps treat hepatitis.

How it works: The Indian trial theorized that yarrow is effective against hepatitis because of the antiseptic action of its tannins, terpeniol, and cineol. Yarrow contains a plethora of chemicals that speed wound healing, including achilletin and achilleine, which encourage blood coagulation. Yarrow also contains azulene, camphor, chamazulene, eugenol, menthol, quercetin, rutin, and salicylic acid, the active ingredient in aspirin. These relieve pain and inflammation.

Who this should benefit: People with hepatitis who have digestive complaints, loss of appetite, and gallbladder problems can all benefit from yarrow.

Who should avoid this: Children, people older than 65, and pregnant or nursing women.

Recommended formulation: Standardized when available.

Usual dosage range: Take a dose of 4.5 g standardized yarrow or 3 g yarrow flowers daily. For infusion, use 1 to 2 teaspoons of dried herb per cup of boiling water. Steep 10 to 15 minutes. Drink no more than 3 cups a day.

Some herbalists recommend external use in the form of a bath using 100 g yarrow per 20 liters of water for all liver disorders.

Time span of therapy: Varies from 1 month to years. The upper limit varies so much because some people must discontinue yarrow when they become sensitized, that is, gradually allergic to the herb.

Side effects: Diarrhea and skin rash, especially if you have a ragweed allergy.

Caveats: Store the herb away from light and moisture. High doses turn urine dark brown.

Other Liver Herbs

ALISMA PLANTAGO-AQUATICA is sometimes called *water plantain* or *mad-dog weed*. The rhizome of this plant contains triterpenes that are poisonous when fresh, so professional processing is a must. Chinese medical practitioners use *A. plantago-aquatica,* which they often call alisma or alismata, in small quantities in concert with other herbs to discourage edema and ascites in hepatitis C. If you are procuring alisma on your own, you should seek out the extract for oral administration or the homeopathic preparations, then take them as labeled.

BUPLEURUM, OR SCUTE. *Bupleurum orfalcatum,* or scutelaria, is called *chái hú* in China. This root member of the parsley family is a widely used Chinese medicine and contains saponin, glycosides, flavonoids, such as the quercetins that may give red wine their cancer-fighting abilities. Scutelaria, or "scute," is thought to increase bile output and to remove toxins and fats. It may also have antiviral properties.

BURDOCK. *Arctium lappa* is called *niú bàng zí* in China and *goboshi* in Japan. Burdock is yet another member of the daisy family. Its roots and seeds contain a veritable cocktail of carbohydrates, vitamins, tannin, and folic acids. Burdock has shown anticancer activity in the test tube because it inactivates cancer-causing agents called *mutagens* (literally "agents of change"). *Arctigenin* in burdock discourages liver-cancer cell growth in test tubes, and as a result, scientists theorize that burdock use is associated with fewer cancerous mutations in cells. There is also clinical evidence for burdock's antibacterial and antifungal action.

The key to using burdock safely is to avoid overdose. Don't use more than ½ to 1 teaspoon of the powder two to three times daily at mealtimes. Use the standardized powdered extract.

PEONY. *Paeonia officinalis,* a plant with beautiful red and white flowers, is widely used for liver diseases, including hepatitis, in Chinese herbal medicine. Peony flowers, dried seeds, and roots reduce the inflammation of hepatitis, due to active ingredients that include *monoterpene ester glucosides, tannins* and *flavonoids.* To make an infusion, steep 1 gram of peony flowers in 1 cup of boiling water for 15 minutes. Drink 1 cup of the infusion daily. The *PDR for Herbal Medicines* reports that there are no health hazards at proper dosages, but some people suffer side effects such as nausea and vomiting.

REISHI MUSHROOMS contain compounds called *triterpenoids* and are touted as liver tonics. Reishi may protect the liver from fibrosis and progression to cirrhosis. These hard woody mushrooms should not be eaten, so the usual method of ingestion is to brew them into a tea. To brew the tea, cut up 3 to 5 grams of the mushrooms, then pour ½ liter boiling water over them, allow to steep for 15 minutes, then drink half the mixture in the morning and half in the evening. Or buy the alcohol extract and take 2 to 3 grams in the morning and 2 to 3 grams in the evening. Up to 10 grams of the alcohol extract a day have been ingested with no reports of toxicity.

SCHISANDRA, *Schisandra chinensis,* is the ripe dried fruit of a vine that is related to the magnolia tree. Lignins and tannins in the herb are thought to reduce liver inflammation, but no scientific tests have yet borne this out. Schisandra is not available in a standardized dosage, but some patent medicines contain 6 to 9 grams; consult a practitioner of traditional Chinese medicine for the correct formulation and dosage.

CH100 is a mixture of nineteen Chinese medicinal herbs in tablet form. It was not yet widely available in the United States as this book went to press, but is being touted as a treatment for hepatitis. This claim cannot be assessed because its formulation has not been revealed. CH100 is now being evaluated in clinical trials in Wales to determine its safety and effectiveness.

Herbs to Avoid

Unfortunately, some herbs do as much to harm your liver as the herbs above do to help. **Ephedra** (*Ephedra sinicia*), or **ma huang** (*E. vulgaris* and other species), has a long history as a Chinese and Asian Indian herb. It was often recommended to treat the symptoms of colds and hay fever. The active ingredients—ephedrine, pseudoepinephrine, and norpseudoepinephrine—are powerful nervous-system stimulants. Because ephedra's active ingredients stimulate the heart, act as a decongestant and open bronchial passages, and increase blood pressure, they appear in FDA-approved over-the-counter medications such as Sudafed.

An *American Journal of Clinical Nutrition* study indicated that ephedra's strong stimulant effect "turns up" your metabolism, resulting in increased weight loss. But it can also cause liver problems. By March 1996 the FDA had released a warning about "Diet Pep," a formulation of ma huang and kola nut that *caused* hepatitis in some users who sought to use it as a liver tonic.

Comfrey, *Symphytum officinale* and *S. uplandicum,* is widely touted as a "general healing agent" when applied topically to sprains and bruises, but people with liver conditions should never take it internally. The *Journal of the National Cancer Institute* revealed that experimental animals developed liver cancer after taking comfrey. *New England Journal of Medicine* relates how a woman washed six daily comfrey capsules down with a quart of comfrey tea, then developed *hepato veno-occlusive disease,* or HVOD, in which the liver's blood vessels narrow dangerously. The herb's pyrroloizidine compounds are also carcinogenic. Canada has banned comfrey.

The FDA says **coltsfoot** (*Tussilago farfara*) is of "undefined safety," but it also contains pyrroloizidines, and the *Journal of the National Cancer Institute* found that animals fed coltsfoot developed liver cancer. Pyrroloizidine in the herbs **borage** and **senecio** also causes liver damage. **"Royal jelly"** is a bee extract that has been billed as a "cure" for liver ailments and insomnia. It has triggered at least ten life-threatening asthma attacks, and *The Medical Journal of Australia* recounts the subsequent death of an asthmatic girl from the potion. People with a history of asthma or other allergic conditions should avoid royal jelly.

Skullcap, also known as Virginia skullcap, Quaker bonnet, hoodwort, helmet flower, and mad-dog weed (not to be confused with Alisma plantago-aquatica, which while sharing a common nickname, is an entirely different herb), whose botanical name is *Scutellaria lateriflora,* causes confusion, giddiness, and severe hepatitis and other liver problems.

In 1992, *Gastroenterology and Clinical Biology* reported that twenty-six people had developed acute hepatitis within nine weeks of taking **wild germander** in an herbal weight-loss concoction. It took many of them half a year to recover. Wild germander has been banned in France.

This is by no means an exhaustive list. **Gordolba yerba, Chinese tea, chaparral, kompocha mushroom, pennyroyal and margosa oils, apiol, *jin bu huan,* mate, tonka beans, melilot, woodruff, vinca, thread-leafed groundsel,** and other herbs also damage the liver. To be sure you have chosen an herb that will help and not harm your liver, be sure to consult your physician before adding any herb to your treatment regimen.

It seems a shame to have to end the chapter on the negative note of herbs that harm the liver, because herbal remedies offer a garden of healing that can ease symptoms and help protect your liver from harm by the hepatitis C virus. And they offer this without the profound fatigue and other side effects of conventional approaches. Just be sure to give herbs the respect they deserve. Recognize them for what they are—powerful medicine—and use them with care.

For more information

Bibliography

Fugh-Berman, Adriane, M.D. *Alternative Medicine: What Works.* Williams & Wilkins, 1997.

Hobbs, Christopher. *Milk Thistle: The Liver Herb.* Botanica Press, 1984.

———. *Foundations of Health: Healing with Herbs and Foods.* Botanica Press, 1992.

Lawrence, Ruth A. and Robert M. Lawrence. *Breastfeeding,* 5th edition. Mosby, 1999. See the "Drugs in Breast Milk" chapter for a comprehensive treatment of herbal medications and breastfeeding.

PDR for Herbal Medicines, 1st edition. Medical Economics, 1999.

Tyler, Varro, Ph.D. *The Honest Herbal.* Haworth Press, 1993.

Organizations

To find an herbalist, contact:

American Association of Acupuncture and Oriental Medicine
    4101 Lake Boone Trail, Suite 201
    Raleigh, NC 27607
    (919) 767-5281
The American Herbalists Guild
    P.O. Box 1683
    Sequel, CA 95073

CHAPTER EIGHT

Taming the Liver's Anger

A light heart lives long.
—*William Shakespeare,*
Love's Labours Lost, Act V, Scene 2

I was once a very calm, unflappable person. Now I'm on an emotional roller coaster, and I know in my heart it has to do with having hepatitis C.

Julie

I'm a nurse, and I know how important your state of mind is to your general health, so I try to stay positive and cheerful.

But when I thought of all the infected people who the government knows are infected but is not telling, when I thought of the fact that there is probably no effective medicine out there for me, when I had to reassure my wife for the tenth time that she is not going to get the virus from me, and tell people for the hundredth time that I didn't get hepatitis from being a drug addict but probably from caring for someone in the hospital, I seemed to stay angry instead.

I knew my anger could cripple my health, so I started going to a support group where I could get these feelings into the open and vent them. Now I find that I don't dwell on them anymore. I'm putting my energy toward getting well, and it's working.

Tom

Hepatitis C and Your Emotions

"In Chinese medical theory, every organ has an emotional component," says Yanqiu He, OMD, L.Ac., of Bethesda, Maryland. "Chinese physicians have held for centuries that the liver is the seat of anger. When the liver has a problem, it leads to emotional changes such as depression and anger." Dr. He is a Doctor of Oriental Medicine and licensed acupuncturist who is board certified in Chinese herbal medicine. She treats hepatitis C patients with a combination of herbs, acupuncture, and Oriental approaches. "The emotional component is very important in hepatitis. In Chinese medicine, the liver is not only the seat of emotions like anger, it is the 'battleground of the body.' " Like many other traditional Chinese medicine practitioners, Dr. He also believes that anger can *cause* liver problems.

Our Western experiences with hepatitis C seem to have borne this observation out. Depression and its traveling partner, fatigue, are an integral part of hepatitis C and other liver diseases.

East and West agree: Positive habits of thought can strengthen your immune system and delay or prevent progression of hepatitis C infection to cirrhosis and liver cancer; negative thoughts can worsen your prognosis. You must improve your emotional and mental state in order to conquer hepatitis C. Western practitioners have amply quantified this mind-body connection. In 1974, University of Rochester psychiatrist Robert Ader created the tongue-twisting specialty of *psychoneuroimmunology* when he illuminated a biochemical link between negative habits of thought and immune-system suppression.

Fortunately, there are many paths to strengthening your liver with your mind. Some of the most important ones are acupuncture, guided imagery, prayer, psychotherapeutic approaches, and support groups, which are described on the following pages.

But first, let's look at the way hepatitis affects the mind.

Depression often accompanies hepatitis. And even people who escape depression are assailed by the profound anxiety of having a disease that is fraught with so much risk and uncertainty. You don't know whether you will be one of the lucky few who clears the virus completely or one of the unlucky few who progresses to severe cirrhosis or liver cancer. You don't know whether the lengthy, difficult, and expensive course of interferon will cure you. Often, you can't even know how you acquired the disease, and you worry about whether you might have transmitted it to a loved one before you learned you had it and were able to take precautions.

Anxiety is especially acute for those few people with hepatitis who need a liver transplant. A 1987 study revealed that the period of liver biopsy and the first signs of organ rejection were described by participants as the most anxiety-producing experiences of their entire lives.

Depression is also a very common side effect of interferon therapy. Interferon-induced depression is made even worse by the fact that common antidepressants, like many other medications, can further harm the liver, and a depressed person may end up having to choose between interferon and antidepressants.

Depression is more than just feeling sad. The negative feelings are overwhelming, persistent, and prevent you from functioning and from enjoying life. If you have any of the signs or symptoms below, please call your doctor for advice, because you may be depressed.

- loss of pleasure in activities you once enjoyed
- loss of appetite for food or sex
- difficulty sleeping, especially if you awaken early in the morning
- feelings of hopelessness
- feelings of worthlessness

Finally, there is the specter of anger, much of it justified in people with hepatitis C. Many people with hepatitis C have shared with me their anger and frustration over the dearth of effective medical treatments. After a long, unpleasant course of medication, most people on interferon relapse after a significant investment of time, money, and emotional upheaval. Like Tom, most people with hepatitis C resent the stigma it carries, even among some physicians and other people who should know better. Because so few people understand the many ways in which it can be transmitted, HCV-infected people must constantly defend themselves against the perceptions that they "must" be drug addicts or alcoholics.

And there is fear. Not just fear for themselves, but as we saw in Chapter 2, the risk of contracting hepatitis C drives a wedge of fear between family members and even between husbands and wives. As a result, the person with hepatitis often feels isolated, shunned, and maligned as an addict and may be totally unaware of how many other people share his or her plight.

As if all this were not enough, the government has not followed through on its earlier commitment to notify the 4 million Americans who are at risk from blood transfusions. Many people learned of their infection by accident only after they had been infected for years. They might have been diagnosed earlier, when chances for a cure and chances to avoid risking the health of others were greater.

Without emotional support and treatment, all this anger can turn inward. Western medicine regards depression and anger as two faces of the same coin, because anger turned inward and directed against the self often manifests as depression. This anger and depression further worsens the health of people who are already under attack by the hepatitis C virus.

The disease itself is stress-inducing. This constant triggering of stress evokes inevitable physical effects, including birth defects, heart attacks, and a decrease in immune-system cells. Although stress is an unavoidable component of life, the stress that makes people sick tends to stem from a condition that the person feels powerless to change. People in high-stress, low-control jobs, such as waiters and assembly line workers, have four to five times as many heart attacks as people with less stress or more control over their situations. You have little control over the stress that hepatitis C creates.

"In Chinese medical theory, long-term anger can damage the liver," adds Dr. He.

So hepatitis C can set a vicious cycle in motion: The assailed liver generates anger. Then, as Tom described so well on page 171, the predicament of the infected person leads to more anger. This can sabotage recovery in many ways:

- Depression and anger worsen the fatigue so common in hepatitis. You may not have the energy to do things that help deal with your disease, such as exercising, eating carefully, attending a support group, and seeking other social psychological support.
- A depressed or angry person may feel frustrated and hopeless and find it harder to stay motivated to comply with the medications and with the nutritional advice of experts.
- A depressed person may need antidepressants to avoid suicidal actions, and antidepressants may further damage his or her liver. He or she may also have to give up interferon, as we saw in Chapter 4.
- Depressed people have weaker immune-system function, so depression can indirectly speed up liver damage and even cirrhosis and cancer.
- There is always the danger that a depressed person will attempt or commit suicide, so depression is a very direct threat to your life as well.

Many doctors find themselves at a loss for medications that can ease symptoms of depression without further endangering the livers of people with HCV, especially people who are taking interferon. In fact, as we saw in Chapter 4, people with uncontrolled depression are rarely prescribed interferon for this reason: Doctors are afraid that discontinuing their patients' psychiatric medications to prescribe interferon may leave them vulnerable to suicidal tendencies.

Many nonpharmacological treatments can help you to disarm the liver's anger and to regain control over the emotional component of hepatitis C. These include lifestyle choices such as drug and alcohol avoidance, and simple steps—rest, stress reduction,

NATURAL ANTIDEPRESSANT OPTONS:
ST. JOHN'S WORT AND SAM-e

Conventional Antidepressant Drugs

Antidepressant drugs can treat and even banish depression, but some have side effects that include liver damage. This is particularly true of older antidepressant drugs, such as the tricyclic antidepressants Elavil and Tofranil (amitriptyline). Their other side effects include drowsiness, blurred vision, weight gain, dry mouth, and constipation. Monoamine oxidase inhibitors (MAOIs) are another type of older antidepressant that includes Nardil and Parnate. These trigger so many interactions that even common foods such as cheese and over-the-counter drugs can cause serious illness or prevent the MAOIs from working. Some psychiatrists prescribe antidepressants to people with hepatitis C, but patients must be monitored closely for side effects and interactions.

The newer antidepressant drugs such as Prozac do not carry the same risk of liver toxicity or other serious side effects. But they can trigger fatigue, insomnia, restlessness, nausea, anxiety, and sexual dysfunction.

Fortunately, there are promising alternatives to prescription drugs that may help people with hepatitis. Although more research is necessary, evidence is mounting that St. John's wort and SAM-e are safe and effective.

St. John's Wort

St. John's wort, or *Hypericum,* contains more than fifty chemicals, and scientist aren't yet sure which is responsible for its demonstrated antidepressant effect. Hyperricin or another chemical in St. John's wort may work as an MAO inhibitor such as Nardil. Or it may work like Prozac by inhibiting the re-uptake of serotonin from neurons in the brain. Or it may increase levels of the neurotransmitters GABA (gamma-amino butyric acid) or dopamine in the brain. St. John's wort may even lift depression by a more subtle route—altering the workings of the immune system.

In *Secrets of St. John's Wort,* Larry Katzenstein describes European studies involving a total of three thousand patients. These studies have established that the herb is as effective as synthetic antidepressants in relieving mild depression. There is no evidence that St. John's wort helps people with serious depression.

A series of U.S. reports published in the 1994 *Journal of Geriatric Psychiatry and Neurology* included seven clinical studies that touted its efficacy. By 1996, St. John's wort had gained the attention of the *British Medical Journal.* Among the thirteen trials it analyzed, six trials found the herb not only superior to placebo but more effective than standard antidepressants in banishing depression. But these were all small trials, so the NIMH (National Institutes of Mental Health) has now undertaken a large double-blind study. ("Double-blind" means that neither the patients nor the doctors know who will receive the substance under investigation and who will get a placebo—"dummy" pill—or another treatment.)

The study in progress for St. John's wort is comparing it with both an antidepressant and a placebo. It is being conducted at Duke University Medical Center in Durham, North Carolina, and Professor of Psychiatry Jonathan Davidson is the principal investigator. Its results won't be in until the fall or winter of the year 2000.

Children and pregnant and breastfeeding women should not take St. John's wort until more is known about its effect on these sensitive populations. Neither should people who are taking prescription antidepressants. People with serious depression should not take St. John's wort, which means that you should see your physician before you take it to make sure that you are not seriously depressed.

There is evidence that St. John's wort makes many fair-skinned people photosensitive, so they should use sunscreen and avoid direct sunlight while taking the herb.

SAM-e

SAM-e (S-adenosyl-methionine) is widely touted as a "natural" antidepressant. SAM-e is sold in Europe mainly as a prescription drug, and has recently been marketed as a supplement in the United States. Richard Brown, a Columbia University psychopharmacologist, and Teodoro Bottiglieri, director of neuropharmacology at Baylor University's Institute for Metabolic Diseases in Dallas, told *USA Today* that they believe SAM-e is "a breakthrough supplement that works as well as prescription drugs [to relive mild depression] in half the time with no side effects."

It is produced by the body, largely in the liver, and plays a number of supportive roles in the body, from maintaining healthy cell membranes to producing key brain chemicals that elevate our mood. Italian doctors routinely prescribe SAM-e as an antidepressant, and a long pedigree of European research has demonstrated its effectiveness and versatility.

One of its most fortunate effects for people with hepatitis C is the fact that it supports liver functioning and self-repair (see Chapter 6).

SAM-e works within days, unlike prescription antidepressants, which commonly require two to three weeks to work optimally. SAM-e seems to be safe, and its most common side effect is gastrointestinal distress. As with St. John's wort, a large-scale, scientifically controlled study in this country is the next step to convincing Americans that SAM-e is an effective antidepressant. As this book went to press, none were yet scheduled for SAM-e.

St. John's wort and SAM-e are not for self-treatment of serious depression. See your physician before you start taking either remedy, because other conditions, such as thyroid dysfunction, can masquerade as depression. And never discontinue a prescription antidepressant abruptly, without consulting your doctor.

exercise—to strengthen the immune system. Herbs, support groups, acupuncture, guided imagery, and last but far from least, prayer, can also play a vital role.

> My depression had been controlled by antidepressants, but it re-turned with a vengeance when I began taking interferon. My doc-tor said that beginning antidepressants again could further harm my liver, so he wanted me to try acupuncture first. I rolled my eyes in response, which was pretty rude, but I didn't believe in that New Age stuff and I felt patronized. "I'll tell you what," he said. "If it doesn't help you, I'll pay for the session—that's how sure I am that you'll benefit from this." Now he had my attention! I am so glad I tried it; it was as if a cloud was lifting. I go regularly and my mood and energy have made a 180-degree turn—without the fogginess and liver damage that a pill would have left me with.
>
> Victoria

Acupuncture

There is ample evidence that acupuncture relieves the stress and also the discomfort of hepatitis C. Acupuncture is a five-thousand-year-old Chinese healing technique that regulates the flow of life energy, or *qi*. In acupuncture, slender needles are in-serted and rotated at specific energy points of the body. These points fall along a dozen different pathways, or *meridians,* that connect vital organs. Stimulation of some of the one-thousand-plus acupuncture points eases pain, releases energy, and stimu-lates the immune system. Very specific patterns of placement have been devised for many illnesses.

Over the past thirty years, copious Western research has veri-fied the effectiveness of acupuncture for pain relief, immune re-sponse, and emotional therapy, all of which are very important in treating hepatitis. In the 1970s, National Institutes of Health researchers Maria Reichmanis, a biophysicist, and Robert Becker, a physician, discovered a parallel between acupuncture points and the body's electrical flow, which they measured by taking the *galvanic skin resistance,* or GSR. They found that the GSR follows the acupuncture meridians. A UCLA study of headache sufferers found that those who underwent acupuncture experienced fewer, less severe episodes of pain. In 1983, the journal *Pain* analyzed several studies and concluded that acupuncture is as effective as Western painkillers.

Dr. He, who is board-certified in herbal medicine and a licensed acupuncturist, believes that the Chinese concept of *qi* explains how acupuncture relieves the symptoms of liver illness. "Acupuncture works by regulating *qi,* which is blocked in hepatitis. Acupuncture is very good at addressing anger, because acupuncture makes *qi* stagnation better; when the *qi* flows more freely, the anger is relieved."

This emotional component is very important in hepatitis because affected people are very depressed and angry due to their liver disease. Acupuncture can loosen this emotional component and make them feel more relaxed. "The Chinese believe that going to a therapist is no good if you don't move the *qi,*" Dr. He says.

"I see a lot of husbands and wives who complain that their infected spouses put them through constant emotional changes," she adds. "I explain, 'It's because of their liver disease; you have got to forgive them.' "

Be sure to choose a licensed acupuncturist, who will, like Dr. He, have the designation L.Ac. appended to his or her title. Your physician or the American Association of Acupuncture and Oriental Medicine can help you find an appropriate practitioner. The address and phone number of that organization are given at the end of this chapter.

If you undergo acupuncture, you will have no more than a dozen points stimulated at any one visit. The sensation will be mildly stimulating, not painful. In this country, most acupuncturists use disposable needles or needles that have been meticulously sterilized. Make sure that yours does; otherwise, needles can spread bloodborne diseases such as hepatitis C. Because needles can't be used on some sensitive points such as the nipple or penis, acupuncturists sometimes practice *moxibustion*. This is the burning of the herb *Artemisa vulgaris,* or *moxa,* above the acupuncture point. Less often, the practitioner may stimulate acupuncture points with lasers, electricity, ultrasound waves, or injections of water or drugs. Be prudent about the latter: Make absolutely sure that the equipment is sterile and find out what is being injected.

In the late 1980s, David Eisenberg, M.D., of Harvard Medical School theorized that acupuncture works by stimulating the release of endorphins, painkilling chemicals released by the brain; these are also released during exercise and are the source of the famous "runner's high." The fact that acupuncture gives pain relief in addition to emotional relief is very fortunate for people with hepatitis C because it allows them to avoid the liver damage that can come with conventional medical pain relievers such as aspirin, indomethacin, and naproxen.

More recent Western medical studies have verified the dramatic relief acupuncture affords for emotional problems as well. In 1992, the Mental Health Center of Waco, Texas, reported that after patients underwent acupuncture, their average hospital stay was reduced from twenty-seven days to eight. Acupuncture made emotionally distressed patients calmer, less confused, and less aggressive, and it fostered better social interaction.

Acupuncture can relieve the nausea of hepatitis C as well. Pressure at a point called the *p-6 neigan,* located about an inch above the wrist, relieved nausea and vomiting for 74 percent of the people in two major studies published in *Acta Anaesthetica Scandinavia* in 1993.

Exercise

Hepatitis C can make you feel so tired that exercise seems the last thing in the world you need. But conventional and alternative practitioners agree: Exercise relieves anxiety, anger, and depression and does wonders for the mental and the physical health of people with HCV. Exercise both prevents and treats depression. It produces the same endorphins that are responsible for the mental benefits of acupuncture. Exercise also helps lower iron levels.

By increasing your feeling of well-being, exercise can emotionally equip you to deal with the disease's frustrations and anxieties. A *Behavioral Medicine* study by J. Griest indicates that when it comes to relieving depression, running works as well as psychotherapy. Working out is such an effective treatment for depression that a 1988 *American Journal of Epidemiology* report by C. E. Ross found that every type of workout decreased anxiety and depression. A study of forty-three women by I. L. McCann found that strenuous exercisers experienced greater relief from their depression than people who used relaxation exercises.

And that's not all. Paradoxically, exercise *relieves* fatigue in many people. A regular workout helps you to recapture some of your old energy.

Finally, exercise is a must for people who want to further reduce their already small chance of developing liver cancer as a result of HCV infection. There is ample evidence that exercise helps keep cancer at bay. For example, a huge NHANES (National Health Nutrition Examination Survey) survey of men found that active men were only half as likely as couch potatoes to develop cancer. Similar research on women tied breast cancer to a sedentary lifestyle.

What type of exercise is best? "Whatever you like and enjoy doing," says Michael Carlston, M.D., a Santa Rosa, California, physician who incorporates exercise into treatment of the persons he treats for hepatitis C. You are more likely to stick to an exercise program that incorporates your favorite sport. Whatever your choice, don't go halfway. Vigorous exercise should be your eventual goal, Carlston says. "My patients with hepatitis C who work out vigorously five times a week do better than the others."

But begin with a physical, and after you have your physician's blessing, start working out gradually, especially if you are older than forty. Begin with a brisk daily walk and build up to whatever you like to do: Don't jump directly into a high-powered exercise program after years of sitting in front of the TV, because that is a prescription for injury. Whether you choose cycling, jogging, basketball, or skating, the trick is to do it at least five times a week for at least thirty to forty-five minutes, being sure to break a sweat. Later, add weight training to your regimen to discourage bone loss. You must be sure to stretch first, then warm up properly. And don't forget to stretch near the end and to end your exercise session gradually, not abruptly. If you feel dizzy, light-headed, short of breath, or exhausted to the point of pain, or if you feel any numbness, slow down—you are doing too much.

Finally, don't think of exercise as exercise. Think in terms of adopting a more active lifestyle. Take the stairs. Take a walk at lunchtime. Meet your friends on the courts rather than in a restaurant. It all adds up to a better mental state and better health.

Guided Imagery

Imagine holding one of your favorite foods, whether it be eggplant Parmesan or a ripe peach, to your nose. Inhale the aroma that wafts to your nostrils, admire the colors, then mentally take a bite.

You probably just released a flow of saliva, and that's what guided imagery is all about. Through guided imagery, you use your imagination to control your biological functions. Scenarios you imagine can control your emotions and directly improve your physical well-being by affecting your physiological responses. At first blush, this sounds like science fiction, but studies have suggested that your imagination can affect your physiology in very specific ways.

Guided imagery illustrates to what extent mental concentration can affect "involuntary" physical functions such as brain wave activity and blood pressure. In this sense, guided imagery is related to other useful techniques such as hypnosis (in which an expert makes suggestions that you incorporate into your behavior) and biofeedback (in which you learn to consciously control "involuntary" functions, using an electronic feedback apparatus). This is a manifestation of the *mind-body connection*.

Examining the brains of people while they are practicing guided imagery is illuminating. *PET* (positron-emission tomography) is a brain-scanning technique that you can think of as a video of a living brain. PET scans taken during guided imagery show brain activity in the visual cortex during visual imagery and in the aural cortex when guided imagery involves hearing something. Many practitioners use *sensory recruitment,* which means they enlist several senses during guided imagery. You practiced sensory recruitment in the example that began this section when you were asked to smell a favorite food, admire its colors, then taste it.

Guided imagery relieves stress. You are probably familiar with the *fight-or-flight* reaction to stress. If you are confronted with a stressful stimulus, your heartbeat increases, your blood pressure soars, you perspire, your digestive tract stops functioning, blood rushes to your legs and arms, and stress hormones such as adrenaline are released to aid either reaction. The stress response involves autonomic responses triggered by the brain centers concerned with breathing, heart rate, and blood pressure as well as the immune system and digestive system. You are ready to fight or run.

All this was very useful to our ancestors, when the stressful stimulus was a charging tiger or a flooding riverbank. But today, when your stress is being caused by a traffic jam, a confrontation with a coworker, or an argument with your wife, this physiological drama does not help. You are all pumped up with nowhere to go. And recurrent stress reactions cause wear and tear on your body and immune system, making you more vulnerable to the ravages of the hepatitis C virus.

Guided imagery reduces this reaction, lowering your breathing rate and blood pressure and lowering the production of "stress hormones." After a single fast, simple training session, you can do it anywhere as often as you feel will help you, with no equipment except your mind.

This simple low-tech approach to stress relief is very effective against emotional stress. We have known since 1974 that it boosts immune-system function in measurable ways as well. In that year, a group of medical students were shown how to practice guided imagery, and the numbers of their secretory IgA cells, an important component of the immune system, skyrocketed.

There are two basic types of guided imagery. In one, called *preconceived,* the healer suggests a specific scenario for you to envision. With the other technique, the healer explains what is going on in your body to cause you problems, and you imagine the scenario that will solve your problem based on your own understanding and visualization of the disease process.

Dr. Michael Carlston prefers this approach. "I encourage people to find their own image. I talk to them, explaining what's going on in their bodies. Then I ask them to imagine healing in their liver. I have them lie down in a quiet space, close their eyes, breathe rhythmically, then see what images come up. It seems to work more powerfully that way." As a simple example, a person taking interferon might imagine the drug as a "smart missile" coursing through her bloodstream to the liver, where it seeks out and destroys the virus. Alternatively, she might imagine milk thistle as a medic on the battlefield that travels from liver cell to liver cell helping to bind up their wounds. Someone who is undergoing chemotherapy or ethanol injection for his liver cancer might imagine the medication shriveling his tumor until it disappears. The scenarios are limited only by your own imagination. What's right is what works for you.

Support Groups

The main goal of a support group is emotional support. This support is very important when you are living with a disease as potentially isolating as hepatitis C. I have attended many support-group meetings and have always been struck by the strong sense of camaraderie. A support group becomes a roomful of best friends who know just how you feel, mentally and physically. You don't have to explain your disease or reassure them about the risk of contracting it. You needn't be defensive about how you acquired it—people in hepatitis C support groups know that all victims of the virus are "innocent."

Confidentiality is sacred in such groups, so you can freely express your doubts and fears without pulling punches. You aren't risking alienating or misunderstanding your fellow members, because they've felt angry, depressed, and frustrated, too.

Besides empathy, a support group also helps foster positive expectations, which can improve your response to treatment. In one study of women with breast cancer, Dr. David Spiegel found that those who joined a support group lived twice as long. Another study of 6,928 adults found that the most socially active people were three times more likely to be alive nine years later.

You will meet people who have lived with the disease for ten, twenty, or forty years and are still healthy or are managing their problems successfully. People who worsen to the extent that they need a liver transplant can meet people who have had transplants and regained their old quality of life. Meeting one such resilient transplant survivor is probably worth more than the verbal assurances of a dozen transplant surgeons. Many people who are cured or who regain their health after a transplant keep attending support groups because they know their presence will help others.

Support groups are also conduits for cutting-edge medical information and treatment tips. Members tend to be sophisticated about the nature and treatment of hepatitis C and eager to share this information with neophytes. You can learn about everything from blood tests to interferon to herbal treatments—nearly every aspect of day-to-day living with HCV. These groups are also invaluable to the newly diagnosed person who is looking for a doctor, nutritionist, or herbalist. Some groups are politically active; others focus more upon the immediate needs of members.

Although support-group members are dedicated to helping each other through this serious health condition, I was struck by how often people laughed and joked. This shared camaraderie often manifested itself as laughter, which is in itself is a very healthy behavior; laughter decreases stress hormones and raises endorphins.

If you have hepatitis C, *please* attend a support group. People often think that only extroverts can benefit from such groups, but they are very beneficial to more private people because they help them to share their emotions and feelings in a safe setting filled with supportive people. So even if you are not a "joiner," the benefits are so dramatic that you owe it to yourself to at least try attending a few meetings.

You owe it to others too, because one of the best things about a support group is that you give and receive *mutual* support. You may meet people in this group who change your life and you may change someone else's.

To find a support group near you, call your local medical center or the American Liver Foundation. If there is no group near you, consider starting one. The free brochure "How to Start a Hepatitis C Support Group" can be obtained from Amgen Corporation or the American Liver Foundation, whose addresses are listed at the end of this chapter.

Prayer

The vast majority of Americans believe in a loving God. All religious faiths stress the powerful impact that a relationship with God can have on the state of your mental and physical health. The power of God to heal people who have not been helped by conventional medicine is a cornerstone belief of all major religions.

I awoke in a hospital bed. For a moment, I forgot where I was and why my hand was bandaged and painful. My husband, André, gently told me, "You became confused yesterday and before I could stop you, you tried to pick up a hot teakettle by gripping the side. You passed out in the ER while we were waiting to have your hand attended to. The doctor says it's the encephalopathy, but he can treat it."

As I lay there, I felt so discouraged. Just when things had been going so well with my new, healthy lifestyle and falling enzyme levels, this had to happen. I began to feel the familiar pangs of anxiety: Was I ever going to get better? André read my thoughts. "It's just a temporary setback," he reassured me.

Just then a rap at the door was followed by a beautiful sight. Everyone from my church study group trooped in, bearing cards, flowers, and fruit. Cyndy, my best friend, clasped my hand, and the others surrounded my bed. "You're going to be fine," she said. "Just to make sure, we're here to pray for you."

By the time they left, I felt happy and at peace. I knew I was going to get well, and I did. And crazy as it sounds, my hand had stopped hurting.

Elaine

Although the news media tend to portray religious and conventional medical approaches as diametrically opposed opposites, this is inaccurate. Over the past decade, medicine has experienced a resurgence of interest in the healing power of prayer. Scientific studies have often confirmed and tried to explain the power of prayer and religious faith to heal. On a purely anecdotal level, many surgeons routinely pray before they go into the operating room.

FAITH'S HEALING POWER.   As we saw at the beginning of this chapter, medical experts agree that positive expectations and emotions about your health can improve your chances of becoming well again. This optimism is analogous to the religious concept of faith.

ATTENDING RELIGIOUS SERVICES.   A report in *Social Science Medicine* analyzed twenty-two studies of people who attended religious services regularly and found that they enjoyed better health. It speculated that people who attend a church, synagogue, or mosque enjoy better health partly because they benefit from the social support they receive.

PRAYING WITH OTHERS.   A study by Randolph Byrd of San Francisco Medical Center, published in the *Journal of the American Medical Association,* found that the "laying on of hands" relieved stress better than drugs. The study also found that patients who were prayed over suffered from fewer complications after surgery. But no convincing scientific benefit has been found for *intercessory prayer,* in which a person or a group of people prays for an absent person.

TWO DISTINCT PRAYING STYLES have been well studied. In *directed prayer,* a person prays for a specific outcome. She may ask for her fibrosis to regress or for liver enzymes to fall back to normal levels. Or she may ask God to clear the HCV from her body altogether.

There is also *nondirected prayer,* in which the supplicant yields himself to God's will, asking God to heal him or asking for a deeper understanding of God's plan for him.

Medical studies theorize that faith and prayer seem to work because they reduce anxiety and because directed prayer works as a sort of guided imagery in which one visualizes healing occurring as a direct result of God's love and mercy.

No studies have suggested that one prayer style is more effective than another, so your beliefs and faith should determine your praying style. Just bear in mind that behavioral adjustment is part of a holistic, spiritual approach to healing. It makes little sense to pray if you continue to eat fatty foods, drink alcohol, live on the couch, and neglect your medications. Spiritual approaches work best when they are a unified part of life, not crisis management.

Psychotherapeutic Approaches

Your hepatitis C infection can create or worsen many psychological issues, as Tom's story illustrated so powerfully at the beginning of this chapter. The suppressed anxiety, anger, and fear caused by the disease can lead to or worsen your depression. Depression, in turn, saps your energy and prevents you from doing the many things you can pursue to make yourself better.

Psychotropic medications taken over a short period of a few weeks help many people conquer their depression. But psychotropic medications may not be a good option for the person with hepatitis C because of the biological stress they place on the liver. Although a relatively undamaged liver can still do its job of metabolizing and excreting the drugs, this extra stress on the liver is unwelcome at a time when you want to give your liver the rest and support it needs to recuperate. Someone whose hepatitis has progressed to fibrosis or cirrhosis can be pushed into further liver damage by daily psychotropic medication. For these reasons, doctors are often reluctant to prescribe medication unless patients are suicidal or unable to function.

There are other drug issues directly related to hepatitis C. If you acquired the virus through drug or alcohol abuse, you must master these problems to control your hepatitis. The best medicines and alternative therapies in the world won't save your liver if you are still drinking or doing drugs. Ask your doctor to refer you to drug counseling or therapy or call Alcoholics Anonymous (1-800-266-5584) or Narcotics Anonymous (1-888-677-8810).

Talk therapy is an important option for people with hepatitis. If you feel overwhelmed by sadness, fear, or anger to the point where you cannot summon the energy to exercise, eat well, or pursue acupuncture or interferon, ask your doctor to refer you to a mental health professional.

If you have begun to feel that your loved ones would be better off without you or if you have fantasies about suicide or homicide, especially fantasies that involve a detailed plan, see your doctor or go to an emergency room immediately—you may be at risk for suicide.

Homeopathy

Homeopathy is the use of minute quantities of pharmaceutically active compounds that have been so heavily diluted that no molecules of the compound remain, only the "impression" of the compound on the molecules of water or alcohol in which it was dissolved. Homeopaths call this "potentization by dilution."

Homeopaths tend to treat symptoms rather than diseases. Their theory adheres to the principle of "like treats like," so to treat a symptom, they use compounds that can cause the same symptom. Symptoms such as hepatitis-related nausea and depression are likely to be treated by a dilution of a compound that would normally trigger nausea and depression or fatigue. Homeopathy uses a variety of treatments for the protection of your liver in early-stage hepatitis. Michael Carlston, M.D., finds that *sulfiuricum, sulfur magnesia,* and *carbonica* are very helpful against the liver damage caused by the virus. Dr. Carlston also uses *nux vomica,* a nut that causes vomiting, in substantial quantities to treat nausea. He uses *cheladonium* to induce better moods and restful sleep. People with severe cirrhosis are often given three to four homeopathic preparations to take every day. These tend be quite specific and tailored to the state of that person's liver. Preparations used in endstage cirrhosis tend to include *c. marianus* and *crotulus hortus,* which stems hemorrhaging.

Homeopathy is considered the practice of medicine, so it can be legally administered only by M.D.'s, D.O.'s (Doctors of Osteopathy), and specially qualified naturopathic physicians (N.D.'s) and chiropractors (D.C.'s). You can buy homeopathic remedies for common medical problems over-the-counter, but I strongly suggest you check with a homeopathic practitioner before doing so.

Herbs

Marcellus A. Walker, M.D., L.Ac., and Kenneth B. Singleton, M.D., M.P.H., recommend the use of prepackaged tinctures of *gotu kola, kava kava,* and *valerian* for relaxation. These herbs soothe without the side effects and liver damage of antidepressant drugs. Take one for four to six weeks according to the package directions. For more about the many uses of herbs in hepatitis C, read Chapter 7, "Herbs."

There are many other alternative approaches to the attainment of inner peace that can also improve your physical health and your ability to withstand the emotional upheaval of hepatitis C. Describing them all is beyond the scope of this book, but there are volumes that do a wonderful job of detailing the many alternative approaches and telling you where to find practitioners and these are listed on page 192.

For more information

Bibliography

Acterberg, Jeanne. *Imagery in Healing: Shamanism and Modern Medicine*. Shambala Publications, 1985.

Benson, Herbert. *The Relaxation Response*. Outlet Books, 1993.

Cousins, Norman. *Head First: The Biology of Hope*. Thorndick Press, 1991.

Eisenberg, David, M.D., and T. L. Wright. *Encounters with Qi: Exploring Chinese Medicine*. Penguin Books, 1987.

Fugh-Berman, Adriane, M.D. *Alternative Medicine: What Works*. Williams & Wilkins, 1997.

Goldberg, Burton. *Alternative Medicine: The Definitive Guide*. Future Medicine Publishing, 1999.

How to Start a Hepatitis C Support Group. Amgen Corporation, Thousand Oaks, California. This free manual is designed to help people with hepatitis C develop a local support group. You may be able to obtain it from the American Liver Foundation.

Locke, Steven, and Douglas Colligan. *The Healer Within*. Mentor Press, 1986.

Panos, Maesimund B., M.D., and Jane Heimlich. *Homeopathic Medicines at Home*. Jeremy Tarcher, 1981.

Organizations

American Association of Acupuncture and Oriental Medicine
4101 Lake Boone Trail, Suite 201
Raleigh, NC 27607
(919) 787-5181

American Liver Foundation
1425 Pompton Avenue
Cedar Grove, NJ 07009-1000

Amgen Corporation
One Amgen Center
Thousand Oaks, CA 91320

National Center for Homeopathic Medicine
801 North Fairfax, Suite 306
Alexandria, VA 22314
(703) 548-7790

The Center For Mind-Body Studies
   65225 Connecticut Avenue, NW, Suite 414
   Washington, DC 20015
   (202) 966-7338
   Fax: (202) 966-2589
Mind-Body Clinic
   New Deaconess Hospital
   Harvard Medical School
   185 Pilgrim Road
   Cambridge, MA 02215
   (617) 632-9530

Physicians
   Yanqiu He, OMD, L.Ac.
   5413 West Cedar Lane, Suite 205C
   Bethesda, MD 20814
   (301) 897-3599

CHAPTER NINE

Putting It All Together

You have nearly come to the end of this book, but not to the end of what you can learn about managing hepatitis C. Most of the information in this chapter also appears earlier in the book, but all the key practical information has been brought together in this one chapter for easy reference. This chapter incorporates information about conventional medicine, diet, exercise, lifestyle, supplements, and herbs into specific practices you can use to craft your own blueprint for living well with hepatitis C. Whether or not you use interferon or ribavirin, your treatment plan will incorporate these prongs of attack:

1. Get an early diagnosis.
2. Make an interferon decision.
3. Devise a dietary strategy.
4. Choose supplements.
5. Choose herbs.
6. Craft a liver-friendly lifestyle.

You can tailor the basic philosophy and elements of the hepatitis C treatment plan to your specific medical profile under your doctor's guidance. The latter portion of this chapter describes successful strategies adopted by practitioners to help people avoid serious illness after acquiring HCV. Here you will read about three people and three treatment programs that have helped them to manage hepatitis C. "Provider profiles" are also interspersed between topics. These capsule profiles of practitioners specify how they blend conventional and alternative approaches.

Get an Early Diagnosis

If you are at risk, get tested right away. You will probably gain the peace of mind of knowing you are not infected. If you are infected, you will be able to start treatment at the point where it is most likely to help you clear the virus. Don't wait for symptoms to appear. They will do so only after your liver has been damaged. Make sure that your ELISA test is confirmed by a RIBA test. Find out what your viral load is, and buy a notebook in which to file all your laboratory tests.

VACCINATION.   As soon as you are diagnosed, get vaccinated against hepatitis A and B. "I'm not a big fan of vaccinations for every illness," says Marcellus Walker, M.D. "But people with HCV fall into a high-risk group for co-infection."

Read Chapter 3 for detailed information that will help you to get an early diagnosis.

Make an Interferon Decision

If you have high viral levels when you are diagnosed, consider beginning interferon right away, because you are statistically more likely to progress to significant liver damage relatively quickly.

If you have low viral levels, consider the fact that the new interferon-ribavirin combinations seem to work especially well for people in the early stages of HCV infection. So seriously think about beginning ribavirin combination treatments now;

discuss it with your doctor. Have your genotype tested to see whether you are in one of the genetic groups (2 or 3) for which interferon works best. Also, have your blood-iron levels tested. As you read in Chapters 5 and 6, high iron levels are associated with poorer outcomes, but your doctor may be able to lower them.

But most of the physicians interviewed for this book said that the person who has low viral levels and wants to try natural remedies has plenty of time to try them first, then proceed to interferon if he or she doesn't see satisfactory results within a few months. To review specific detailed information that will help you decide whether interferon therapy or other conventional medical approaches are for you, read Chapter 4.

Devise a Dietary Strategy

Diet is an important part of your treatment plan. Here are foods you should seek out and foods you should avoid if you have hepatitis C.

VEGETABLES
Number of servings: Five a day.

Most vegetables, especially fresh or cooked onions, beets, asparagus, artichokes, and leafy dark-green vegetables. Also, bell peppers, tomatoes, avocados, leeks, celery, watercress, water chestnuts, scallions, snow peas, cauliflower, broccoli, potatoes, yams, sweet potatoes, cabbage, lettuce, and zucchini. Limited servings (one to two daily) of whole vegetable juices are beneficial, especially unprocessed fresh carrot and beet juices.

FRUIT
Number of servings: Five a day.

Most fruits, especially lemons, grapefruits, limes. Also, oranges, apples, raisins, grapes, mangoes, papayas, plums, cherries, raspberries, apples, apricots, figs, melons, peaches, pears, passion fruit, berries, and black currants.

Avoid bananas and persimmons because of their very high sugar content.

NUTS AND SEEDS
Number of servings: Two a day.

Sunflower seeds, walnuts, soybeans, sesame seeds, black currant seeds, pumpkin seeds, peanuts, pecans, almonds, and cashews.

OMEGA-3 OILS
Number of servings: Three a week (five a week if you eat no poultry).

Salmon, mackerel, tuna, bass, rainbow trout, herring, soybean oil, sesame oil, linoleic acids, olive oil, canola oil.

WHOLE GRAINS
Number of servings: Four a day.

Oat bran, oatmeal, brown rice, buckwheat, bulgur wheat, whole-grain breads, müesli.

POULTRY
Number of servings: Two to three a week (optional).

Turkey (preferably free-range), chicken, egg whites.

BEANS
Number of servings: Two to three a day.

Kidney beans, great northern beans, lentils, adzuki beans, tofu, sprouts, mung beans, chickpeas, butter beans, black-eyed peas, peas, baby lima beans.

DIETARY HERBS AND SPICES
Turmeric and garlic should be used at least once a day; also shiitake mushrooms, ginger, and basil.

WATER
Number of servings: Eight to ten glasses of filtered or purified spring water a day.

Drink one glass a half hour after breakfast and one glass between breakfast and lunch, one glass a half hour after lunch and one glass between lunch and dinner, one glass a half hour after dinner and an additional glass while exercising. Then drink two glasses before bedtime. Drink 5 ounces of water with meals, but omit this water if you are suffering from nausea.

LIMIT THESE FOODS
- salt (including salted snacks, soy sauces, and MSG)
- sugar
- drinks other than water and fruit juices

AVOID THESE FOODS COMPLETELY
- alcohol
- dairy products of any kind
- processed and preserved take-out foods
- caffeine
- red meat
- raw seafood such as sushi, mussels, or clams
- chocolate
- coconut oil, palm oil
- artificial sweeteners

INTERFERON MODIFICATIONS
Drink at least ten glasses of water daily.

ADDITIONAL RESTRICTIONS FOR PEOPLE WITH CIRRHOSIS OR LIVER CANCER
- no chicken
- no pork, especially ham, bacon, and salami
- no gelatin

Chapter 5 gives very detailed information about how specific foods and nutrients can bolster your overall health, maintain your liver's function and regenerative powers, and support your immune system.

Choose Supplements

Kenneth B. Singleton, M.D., and most other physicians who use complementary approaches to treat hepatitis C administer large doses of vitamin C intravenously to bolster their patients' immune systems. Pycnogenol (pine bark or grapeseed extract); omega-3 oils that reduce inflammation; colostrum; and transfer factor are even more powerful antioxidants than vitamin E and vitamin C. Coenzyme Q-10 also works well to modulate your immune system. If your liver disease has progressed beyond stage 2, B-complex vitamins, selenium, zinc, magnesium, and calcium are especially important. UltraClear can also help to detoxify a moderately damaged liver.

TO REDUCE YOUR LIVER-CANCER RISK. These nutritional supplements reduce your chances of progressing to cancer: 400 to 800 IU daily of vitamin E; 200 to 300 micrograms daily of selenium; 500 milligrams of vitamin C four to five times a day (after a blood-iron test and if your doctor approves); 50 milligrams a day of coenzyme Q-10; 3 milligrams daily of copper; 15 milligrams daily of zinc; and 250 to 500 milligrams daily of the amino acid l-cysteine.

For detailed information on which specific supplements, in which amounts, can help you in your battle with hepatitis C, see Chapter 6.

Choose Herbs

Herbs are powerful agents that help you quell hepatitis C symptoms by cleansing and supporting the liver and immune system. Dandelion root and milk thistle clean the liver effectively, but their action is so strong that people sometimes experience side effects such as dizziness and headache. Buplerum, or scutelaria, is a very effective alternative. So are licorice, astragalus, schisandra, artichoke, golden seal, reishi and even shiitake mushrooms.

If you visit a practitioner of Oriental medical such as Yanqiu He, OMD, L.Ac., who practices in Baltimore, Maryland, you will be given different herbs in combinations rather than singly. Peony, very small amounts of burdock, and alismatis are popular in Chinese practice. The combinations usually include some scutelaria, or buplerum, but the mixtures change as your liver health changes. However, if you are taking interferon, you usually should not take buplerum or licorice as well: Both affect the metabolism of interferon and can cause overdoses.

For more information, see Chapter 7, which offers very detailed information on a variety of herbs that bolster liver function and actually help to restore the liver's function and health. It gives important information about proper regimens for taking herbs, with information on preferred formulations, dosing, interactions, and even which herbs have been demonstrated to cause liver problems.

Craft a Liver-Friendly Lifestyle

EXERCISE.   Begin exercising to build stamina and to relieve fatigue and stress. If you are a couch potato, see your physician first for the green light, then start slowly. Walk, take the stairs instead of the escalator, invest in a treadmill to walk while you watch TV. Build up to as vigorous a level as possible. Jog, cycle, and do weight training, which is especially important to help perimenopausal women avoid bone loss, between three and five times a week.

You may have to eventually take your activity level down a peg because interferon therapy or hepatitis C itself may sap some of your energy as the disease progresses. But try for forty minutes of vigorous activity five times week. And don't forget to warm up and stretch.

JOIN A SUPPORT GROUP.   You absolutely should try attending a support group. Such a group may be the single most important advantage you acquire in your mental struggle against hepatitis C. Many people initially reject the idea because they envision a pity party where people spend all their time sobbing on each others' shoulders. People do cry sometimes, and it is healthier than crying alone. But a support group is so much more than that. It is an invaluable source of support, treatment information, advice, and tips that make the disease easier to live with. You will also make a roomful of friends who know exactly what you are going through.

PROVIDER PROFILE:
P. LOUNETTE HUMPRHREY, M.D.

Dr. Humphrey is a psychiatrist on the clinical faculty at the Louisville School of Medicine Department of Psychiatry in Louisville, Kentucky. She runs a support group for hepatitis C patients with a colleague, Barbara Miller, R.N., MSN. The telephone number is (502) 852-5867.

Words to Live By
"The more angst someone is feeling over the diagnosis of hepatitis C, the better the support-group experience is for them."

PRAY OR MEDITATE. At the earliest stages, there are many things you do not know about your illness. For most people, the progression to liver damage takes place very slowly, but for a very few, it happens relatively quickly. You do not know whether you will be one of those unlucky few or whether you will ever develop extensive cirrhosis or liver cancer. For this reason, many people choose to pray in a nonspecific manner, asking God to heal them, to give them the wisdom to make the right treatment and lifestyle choices, and to prepare them for what they will undergo.

BEGIN PRACTICING VISUAL IMAGERY. Based on what you have learned about the disease, imagine your liver locked in a life-and-death struggle in which it is holding its own. Develop you own "script," but consider a scenario in which liver cells throw off the invading virus, then clear the virus completely from your body.

ACUPUNCTURE. Acupuncture treatments from two to four times a month relieve stress, pain, and much of the discomfort associated with hepatitis C. "The liver is the center of anger and frustration in the Oriental medical scheme," muses Dr. Marcellus A. Walker, a physician and licensed acupuncturist. "But when it is balanced, the liver is the great harmonizer. Acupuncture helps people achieve that balance."

HOMEOPATHY. Homeopathy uses a variety of treatments for the protection of your liver in early-stage hepatitis. Michael Carlston, M.D., often uses *sulfiuricum, sulfur magnesia,* and *carbonica* to fight against the liver damage caused by the virus. Other remedies work well against common symptoms of hepatitis C, such as *nux vomica,* which controls nausea. People with severe cirrhosis are usually given three to four homeopathic preparations to take every day.

PROVIDER PROFILE: MICHAEL CARLSTON, M.D.

914 Airway Court, Suite 14
Santa Rosa, CA 95403
(707) 545-1554
Fax (707) 545-1595

Dr. Carlston uses a mixture of homeopathy, diet, and conventional treatment to help people with hepatitis C.

Words to Live By
"A patient's health and life are his or her responsibility, and I don't feel I am here to tell them precisely what to do. I lay out facts and help patients to interpret them according to their specific needs. I encourage some people to try more conventional approaches; to others I say, 'Consider an alternative first.' "

To learn more, read Chapter 8, which gives scientific explanations of the mind-body connection. It also offers many more details and specific techniques of strategies that can reduce stress and enhance your mental resiliance.

Three Patients, Three Treatments

The rest of this chapter is devoted to illustrating how three patients at different stages of hepatitis C and with different needs integrate conventional and alternative treatments to meet their health goals.

Art is a forty-seven-year-old health worker who has early-stage hepatitis C. He has little liver damage and does not want to pursue interferon therapy. David, age sixty, is a writer with severe cirrhosis. He is seeking a treatment program that will lend support to his interferon therapy. Zora is a thirty-five-year-old African-American woman who was recently diagnosed with hepatitis C. She wants to treat her hepatitis C with natural approaches and to recapture her earlier energy level. Their names and some details have been changed to protect their confidentiality, but their successes are real. I suggest that you read their stories with an eye toward gleaning what you think might work for you, then discussing it with your physician and other health care providers. I hope you will derive not only knowledge, but also inspiration.

Art

ART'S LIVER-SUPPORT PROGRAM

Eliminate alcohol

Liver-friendly diet

Supplements

Herbs

Homeopathy

Treadmill, cycling, and weight training

Support group

Arthur, or as he prefers to be called, Art, is divorced and lives in the heart of the Poconos. He's forty-seven, but he looks ten years younger, thanks to good genes and a health-conscious lifestyle. He has thick red hair, blue eyes, and a muscular build, and his upbeat, generous nature makes him popular at the emergency room where he works as a physician's assistant. Art exercises daily, running on the treadmill in the hospital gym. He runs, hikes, and cycles on his days off and ran the Boston marathon in 1993. Art often self-treated his colds and minor illnesses with over-the-counter homeopathic remedies. "I believe in conventional medicine, of course, otherwise I wouldn't be a P.A. But I prefer to try milder, safer remedies before I pull out the big guns of pharmaceuticals. However, in retrospect, some of those flulike illnesses I treated with homeopathic remedies were probably symptoms of HCV infection that I never recognized."

In May 1995, Art decided to give blood. "It was a spur-of-the-moment thing, but it probably saved my health. I was riding my bike past a blood drive, and I just stopped."

Diagnosis

Three weeks later, a letter from the blood bank informed Art that he was infected with HCV. He called his doctor, Marcellus Walker, M.D., L.Ac., who tested him again on July 15.

Art's ELISA was positive for HCV. "But I once had an experience with another healthy hospital worker whose ELISA test was also positive for HCV," recalls Dr. Walker. "When I administered a more specific test, that woman turned out not to have the virus after all. A person whose ELISA is positive for hepatitis C always needs to confirm the presence of HCV with a RIBA test." The RIBA confirmed that Art did have hepatitis C. Dr. Walker then determined Art's viral load with a RNA-PCR test. It was relatively low, which was good news. People with low viral loads are more likely to clear the virus from their bodies, and they respond better to interferon or ribavirin therapy. "I track the viral load over time, because it is important to know whether therapy is effective and beneficial," adds Dr. Walker.

PROVIDER PROFILE:
MARCELLUS WALKER, M.D., L.Ac.

1-888-ANTI AGE
Web site: www.aahealth.com

Dr. Walker is the founder of a multidisciplinary group practice in
New Windsor, New York. He is also the medical director of the
Wayne Woodland Manor in Pennsylvania. Dr. Walker is an
herbalist and licensed acupuncturist who holds a master's degree
in spiritual psychology, and uses all these modalities and others
to treat people with hepatitis C.

Words to Live By
"Conventional medicine suppresses; alternative medicine builds
up. You may be suppressing the virus with medications, but what
are you doing to upgrade your immune and digestive systems?"

Art had never had a blood transfusion. He had smoked mari-
juana and had been a weekend binge drinker in college, where he
had experimented briefly with snorting cocaine. "But I cleaned
up my act twenty-five years ago. I've never used IV drugs." Art
did not recall ever being stuck with a needle at work, and his low
viral load argued against his having been infected through a needle stick. Art had no piercings, tattoos, or history of medical care
abroad. Art's was one of the 40 percent of hepatitis C cases
whose origins are unclear.

Dr. Walker scheduled a biopsy to learn more about how hepatitis C had already affected Art's liver and to serve as a baseline.
He also scheduled a slew of diagnostic tests to see how hepatitis C
had affected Art's liver.

Dr. Walker ended their first session by giving Art a selection of
publications that explained hepatitis C treatment options, including information on herbs, supplements, interferon, and ribavirin. "I told Art to study these because after his diagnostic tests

were completed, we would be discussing treatment decisions. This time, *he* is the patient."

Art spent the rest of the month in a diagnostic whirl that started with an ultrasound test, followed by a CT scan and a slew of blood tests. "Luckily, I worked at the hospital where my tests were being done, so I could easily integrate my two roles of caregiver and human pincushion," Art says, laughing. "I spent a lot of time running between the ER and the clinical labs." During this time, Art monitored his symptoms carefully and noted that he suffered from fatigue, vague aches and pains, and almost continuous digestive upset. He often experienced constipation, diarrhea, gas, and belching.

Art decided to tell his coworkers he was infected because "I have a responsibility to my patients. My boss and I sat down with the hospital's top infection-control officer, and we determined that I could safely do invasive procedures if I took additional precautions. My colleagues were wonderful. No one treated me any differently. That was a big load off my mind."

Monitoring Tests

At the beginning of August, even while some of the liver-function tests were still being evaluated, Dr. Walker met with Art to discuss general treatment options. "But first, I want to understand how my patients *feel,*" says Dr. Walker. "Art felt tired, but he couldn't sleep through the night. And he often felt bloated, gassy, and sometimes nauseous."

When Art returned to Dr. Walker's office a week later, he learned that his liver revealed no signs of fibrosis and his blood cell counts were within the normal ranges. But his ALT and other liver enzyme levels were slightly above normal. Under the microscope, his biopsy sample had revealed some areas of inflammation. He was in stage 1, "the second-best possible state of liver health for someone with chronic hepatitis," Art says.

But his genotype was not good news. Art's geneotype was 1a, which has the poorest track record for improvement on interferon therapy.

Art's Treatment Strategy

As a medical worker, Art already knew that hepatitis C was probably not going to kill or cripple him. But he was worried about how best to keep his liver inflammation from progressing. The first major strategy decision was whether they would try to eradicate the virus with interferon.

"In the early phase, I'm not convinced that a person needs interferon," says Dr. Walker. "Art had little evidence of liver inflammation, so I suggested we start his treatment from a nutritional point of view."

For his part, Art was adamantly against using interferon first. "I don't want to feel more tired. I don't want to risk depression and all the side effects. I feel I have plenty of time to fall back to interferon if nothing else works." Dr. Walker devised a treatment plan of diet, supplements, and herbs. His strategy was to support the digestive function of Art's liver, to enhance his immune system, and to treat symptoms that could erode Art's quality of life.

Exercise

Art was already physically active, and during this initial strategy meeting, Dr. Walker advised him that even if his fatigue worsened, he should try to work out three times a week. Workouts would bolster his immune system, relieve stress, and maintain his sense of control over his life. "Just try and stop me," Art replied. Dr. Walker also suggested Art try a support group. "I'm not much of a joiner," Art told him. "Take the phone number anyway," suggested Dr. Walker. "You might change your mind."

Diet

Dr. Walker explained to Art that supporting the liver's digestive functioning was the first priority. He told Art that the digestive stress caused by his infection had to be resolved before the liver would begin to detoxify itself. "The liver won't dump toxins into an inflamed gut; it holds back. So first I want to resolve the problems of constipation, diarrhea, gas, and belching. As these get better, the liver will drain bile and be less stressed. The liver can then start to detoxify itself. When it can again regulate hormones and proteins and eliminate toxins, it will begin clearing the HCV from your body."

Art ate a varied diet that included dairy products, beef, and pork. He also enjoyed a glass or two of wine and high-calorie desserts with dinner on weekends. His three-cup-a-day coffee habit fueled late-night hospital shifts.

Dr. Walker immediately banned the alcohol, dairy products, meats, coffee, and fried foods. He limited Art's salt consumption to two teaspoonfuls a day and told him to stop buying processed foods and to start cooking his own from fresh ingredients. Dr. Walker put Art on a diet that incorporated only organic natural foods, "free of pesticides that can tax the liver." Art's new diet emphasized cooked vegetables and cooked grains. Nuts and seeds provided fatty acids from plant sources. Art ate oatmeal or cooked low-fat müesli for breakfast and ate kasha or unprocessed brown rice as side dishes. He also ate salmon, mackerel, and tuna three times a week, which provided protein and the omega-3 fish oils that can cut inflammation.

Supplements

Dr. Walker replaced Art's multivitamin with an iron-free food-based multi and a 400-milligram **folic acid** supplement. He also prescribed 2,000-milligram vitamin C supplements, alpha-lipoic acid for liver detoxification, and **coenzyme Q-10** for protein production.

Herbs

Then Dr. Walker also recommended the herb golden seal. "It works as a natural anti-inflammatory that also improves immune-system function. If we don't see lower liver enzymes in two months, I will add other supplements with stronger detoxifying and immune-support function."

Psychological Support

Art faithfully adhered to the diet for a month. He had less fatigue and better-quality sleep and his digestive upsets disap-

peared. But he noticed that when he was under stress, his digestive, sleep, and fatigue problems would return briefly. "That's
not unusual," said Dr. Walker. "The liver and the emotions are
closely intertwined; that's one reason why I suggested the support group. But there are other things you can do. Here, have
a seat."

In five minutes, Dr. Walker showed Art the technique of
guided imagery. Art leaned back in his chair and imagined his
immune-system cells as guided missiles that were targeting the
virus instead of his own liver cells. "Guided imagery helped me.
I no longer got sick when I felt stressed."

A week later, Art was disappointed to learn that his liver tests
had not changed. Dr. Walker was reassuring, reminding Art that
"it's really too early to expect to see improvement."

"I knew he was right," recalls Art, "but I couldn't help feeling
discouraged. I knew intellectually that ALT levels fluctuate even
as your liver is recovering, but that didn't ease my deep disap-
pointment. I went home that night and realized that I was depressed. I had been so disciplined, working out when I was 'too
tired,' passing up dessert, eating beets, which I hate, and taking
handfuls of pills. I was feeling sorry for myself.

"And scared. What if the nutritional approach didn't work?
Would anything work? As my heart begin to pound, I reflexively
leaned back and began practicing guided imagery. Suddenly, I
knew what I needed: I needed to talk to someone who had made
it through this."

Art called the number of the support group. "To make a long
story short, it has been a lifeline. I go every other Saturday afternoon, and now I know many people who have gotten well after
disappointing test results."

Art also tried acupuncture with good results. "The support
group helped my outlook, but part of me used to stay angry until
I tried acupuncture," Art admits. "I don't feel sick, but I can't run
marathons now. I can't do invasive procedures on patients without worrying about an accident. The acupuncture helps handle
the curves that hepatitis throws my way."

More Supplements

Dr. Walker had Art add the supplements pycnogenol (pine bark), N-acetylcysteine, a sulfur-based amino acid, and SAM-e, which increases ATP (adenosine triphosphate), the body's energy-pumping system. He also recommended the herb scutelaria.

Success

In December, Art's ALT levels fell to normal levels and stayed there.

In January, six months after he had been diagnosed, Art started the New Year off right with a biopsy that showed that his liver inflammation had decreased. His liver was healing itself.

Five years later, Art maintains his hepatitis treatment plan and has no symptoms aside from mild fatigue. "It sounds ironic, but I'm healthier today than I was before I was diagnosed. I eat better, feel better, and my emotional state is miles better, thanks to guided imagery and my support group. Today, I have a better life, and sometimes I think I owe it all to hepatitis C."

PROVIDER PROFILE: STEVEN J. BOCK, M.D.

Rhinebeck Health Center
Rhinebeck, NY
(914) 876-7082
and Center for Progressive Medicine
Albany, NY
(518) 545-0082

Dr. Bock is the cofounder of two health centers in upstate New York: the Rhinebeck Health Center and the Center for Progressive Medicine in Albany. He is also a founder of patientsamerica. com, a patient-advocacy Web site.

Expertise
Dr. Bock uses a variety of treatment modalities, including preventive, nutritional, and herbal medicine and acupuncture to

help people with hepatitis C. He is board-certified in family practice, certified in acupuncture, and a Diplomate of the American Academy of Anti-Aging Medicine.

Words to Live By
"I practice progressive medicine, which blends the best of conventional medicine and alternative medicine, using an alternative approach to each individual patient."

David

DAVID'S LIVER-TREATMENT PROGRAM

Interferon

Eliminate nicotine and caffeine

Eliminate excess dietary fat and animal protein

Liver-friendly diet

Supplements

Herbs

Homeopathy

Regular mild exercise

David is a sixty-year-old writer who was diagnosed with hepatitis C in 1989. He thinks he was infected by a blood transfusion in 1977, but didn't feel sick until the late 1980s. Before seeing Dr. Bock, David had been taking interferon for a month. "I hated the side effects," says David. "It kept my liver from deteriorating further, but I still felt like hell. A woman in my support group said that Dr. Bock's unique approach had helped her become energetic and symptom free. So I made an appointment. When I first saw Dr. Bock, he asked me what symptoms I had and I said 'All of them, I think.' I was constantly exhausted, I was jaundiced, and I suffered from encephalopathy that made me confused sometimes. In a way, that was the worst; I had been a journalist before I got sick, and I didn't like the lack of focus and control that came with the 'brain fog.' I worried that it might become permanent."

David's Interferon-Support Strategy

"When I first saw David, he looked considerably older than his sixty years," recalls Dr. Bock. "His skin color was a dull ashen gray with a yellowish cast. He was short of breath after walking the few steps from the waiting room to my office. He seemed a little unfocused and his wife had to prompt him often so he could answer my questions. David is a pleasant person, but he seemed unhappy. I explained to him that I take the best of alternative and conventional medicine: I use a progressive approach and this has allowed me to help people with hepatitis C dramatically improve their health and quality of life." Dr. Bock further explained to David that for people with more serious liver damage, he finds that a treatment plan incorporating conventional approaches works best. "As your cirrhosis progresses, the changes in your body become more dramatic. Liver scarring leads to mitotic changes in the cells and increases the risks of liver cancer. You need stronger treatments and must use more conventional treatments." But even in advanced cases such as David's, Dr. Bock takes an integrative approach. "Interferon can reduce liver enzymes and diuretics can banish ascites, but I also provide nutritional and immune-system support. I put David on an interferon-ribavirin modified program."

Diet

First, Dr. Bock discussed David's diet with him; it was poor by any standards. Dr. Bock explained that neither interferon nor alternative treatment would help David if he didn't adopt a diet that gave his liver a fighting chance. Dr. Bock listed the things David would have to cut out of his life altogether: He drank three or four cups of coffee a day as a pick-me-up when he felt especially tired. What's more, David smoked a pipe. He had cut down to one pipeful a day, but that was not enough: He would have to quit altogether—now. Dr. Bock recommended acupuncture treatments to help him. David was to use no sugar, preservatives, or chemical additives. He was to eat only organic foods.

David took a daily multivitamin but ate few vegetables. Fortunately, he liked fresh fruit and ate it three or four times a day. David's cirrhosis was robbing him of his appetite, and he was eating very irregularly. He had long ago fallen into a pattern of eating only his favorite foods. Unfortunately, these were things like fried chicken, grilled-cheese sandwiches, and pizza. But his cirrhotic liver could no longer tolerate such fatty foods, and he was often violently nauseous. "His diet was a huge part of Dave's problem, and I spent much of that first hour doing nutritional counseling. I explained that his fondness for chicken had a lot to do with the encephalopathy that worried him so much. That seemed to get his attention. He began eagerly quizzing me about the foods that would help him feel best."

Dr. Bock put David on a diet that excluded dairy products, including his beloved grilled-cheese sandwiches. Bock suggested sandwiches made of whole-grain bread and soy-milk "cheese" instead. Instead of meat and chicken, David was to eat mostly vegetable protein from veggies, nuts, and seeds. He could have deep-sea fish three to five times weekly, but most of his meals were to consist of vegetables, especially greens, asparagus, onions, and beets. He was to try to eat five servings daily of unprocessed low-sugar fruits such as tangerines. "I explained to David's wife how important it is to shop in organic markets, to cook Dave's food with very little fat and sugar, and to avoid processed and take-out foods like the plague. And I replaced his supermarket multivitamin with a food-based organic brand."

By the second visit, David had given away his pipe, switched to decaf coffee, and stopped eating chicken and dairy. But he was still struggling with his diet. "I admitted to Dr. Bock I still sneaked the occasional burger, but less often than at first. My wife is a great help. She does the shopping, which is no mean feat because she drives miles out of her way to buy organic produce and seafood for me. It's so hard to find foods without added fat and sugar. And she eats only what I can eat; that helps a lot."

Supplements

At their second meeting, Dr. Bock drew David's blood and performed a series of blood tests that revealed that Dave had very low levels of key immune-system and anticancer agents. For example, his DHEA and insulin growth hormone levels were very low. DHEA is an intermediary steroid hormone that is anabolic. That is to say, it builds up reserves of necessary substances, in this case, anticarcinogenic and antistress agents. "These biomarkers indicated that to bolster Dave's immune system and to protect him against cancer, David needed antioxidants badly. So I administered an intravenous injection of vitamin C, and I also gave him B-complex vitamins, glutathione lipoic acid, and thymic extract.

"When I saw David three weeks later, his muscle tone and stamina had begun to return. He was no longer out of breath and he smiled often. My physical examination revealed that David was much better. But his liver enzymes indicated that his cirrhosis was still progressing. I administered a large dose of transfer factor, a food supplement that works by transferring an immune recognition from one person to another, and suggested that he take a smaller maintenence dose daily until his next visit." Transfer helps to treat long-term infections such as hepatitis C. (See Chapter 6.)

"What if this doesn't help me further?" David asked.

"There are many things we can try next, including N-acetyl-cysteine, alpha-lipoic acid, and SAM-e," said Dr. Bock. "But let's give the transfer factor and other supplements a little time to work first."

Herbs

Dave's next visit took place a month after his first session with Dr. Bock, and he had some successes to report. "I'm sticking religiously to my new diet, and I'm even having fun with it. My wife and I have begun creating healthful versions of my favorite foods. She made a tofu dish with sesame sauce that tastes a lot like General Tso's Chicken, a take-out favorite of mine. She started showing me how to cook liver-healthy foods with herbs and seasonings that make them fat-free yet still tasty; I've discovered that I kind of get a kick out of cooking, and now I'm doing my share."

Then Dr. Bock and David talked about herbs. David had always wanted to try milk thistle, but his hepatologist had dismissed herbs as "worthless." Dr. Bock explained that the silymarin in milk thistle does protect the liver, and that scutelaria, buplerum, and licorice are also beneficial. But he prescribed a different herb, astragalus, for David, because it would provide immune-system stimulation for Dave's more advanced disease. Dr. Bock also recommended that David use shiitake mushrooms to protect against cancer, adding, "Now that you're a chef, you can try cooking with them."

At the next visit three weeks later, "David looked like a different person from the one who had barely been able to walk into my office less than two months earlier. He still has cirrhosis, but his encephalopathy has disappeared, he can tolerate mild exercise, his jaundice has abated somewhat, and his liver enzymes are down. He is no longer depressed. David continues on interferon and he is still taking supplements."

David's course of interferon may or may not clear the virus from his system, but his chances of a cure and his quality of life have been considerably improved by his new diet and the immune-system support rendered by the supplements. Thanks to progressive medicine, David has hope again.

Zora

ZORA'S LIVER-PROTECTIVE PROGRAM

Liver-friendly diet

Toxin avoidance

Running, swimming, water aerobics, weight training

Supplements

Herbs

Prayer, guided imagery, support-group meetings

Zora is a thirty-five-year-old freelance graphic artist who found out she was infected with HCV in March 1997. She had undergone a battery of tests to find out why she had developed intermittent flulike symptoms and had grown too fatigued to keep up her rigorous exercise program. After five months of seeing specialist after specialist, diagnostic tests revealed she had hepatitis C. Her symptoms worsened considerably after she moved from a suburb of Seattle to New York City in early June. Zora did not know how she might have contracted the virus. She had never used drugs, although she often drank a glass or two of wine with dinner. She had lived in Gabon for two years while serving in the Peace Corps, and in Rimes, France, for one year, but doesn't remember ever having had surgery or invasive procedures. She did have acupuncture during her stay in France, and this might have been performed with improperly cleaned needles. Also, she had gotten a small tattoo in 1996, so she might have acquired HCV from tainted tattoo needles.

Whatever its origin, hepatitis C was threatening to turn Zora's life upside down. "I was a sprinter in college, and captain of the Georgetown women's basketball team," says Zora. "Until a month ago, I still ran and swam nearly every day, and the idea of having to abandon my workout program frightens me; it's such a big part of who I am. What was I going to do instead, watch TV and play bingo? Physical activity boosts my self-esteem, keeps me in shape, and keeps me emotionally balanced better than psychotherapy ever could. I had to beat this thing. Fortunately, my viral load was low, and I was told that this increased my chances of emerging without serious permanent liver damage.

"But I didn't know what to do. Should I use interferon? I preferred to try a natural approach first: I didn't like what I had read about the debilitating fatigue and other side effects. Although I knew it was a small risk, I was concerned about the fact that interferon increases one's risk of vitiligo. Because I have two cousins and a brother with the disorder, I felt I was already at high risk. Because I am African American, the loss of skin color would be much more noticeable than it is in whites. It can be really disfiguring.

PROVIDER PROFILE:
KENNETH B. SINGLETON, M.D., M.P.H.

Office: (410) 296-3737

Dr. Singleton is clinical assistant professor of medicine at Howard University College of Medicine in Washington, D.C. He uses a blend of conventional, herbal, nutritional, and other complementary approaches to treat hepatitis C patients. Dr. Singleton and Dr. Marcellus Walker are the co-authors of *Natural Health for African Americans*.

Words to Live By
"Find a physician who is knowledgeable about treating hepatitis C—that should be your number-one act."

"But did I have time to pursue a natural approach? I had done a lot of reading about the disease, and some magazine articles suggested that interferon was my only chance to escape severe cirrhosis and liver cancer. I didn't want my interferon window of opportunity to close on me. I looked up a hepatitis C support group. During the 'announcements' period, I told the members that I was looking for a doctor and passed around my notebook asking people to write down the names of doctors they could recommend. Of the seven people who wrote suggestions, two of them had suggested Dr. Singleton. So I called him first."

Zora's Strategy Meeting

"My first impression of Zora was of a young woman who takes care of herself," said Dr. Singleton. "She is a tall, slender but muscular woman who still looks like the captain of a basketball team, with glowing skin and confident movements. Zora strode into my office holding a sheaf of hepatitis C articles, a copy of her laboratory reports, and a small notebook on which she had written a series of question. Right then, I knew that she had already taken the first steps toward healing: She had found a physician-advocate and she had educated herself. I examined Zora's lab work and drew blood for additional tests. Zora had a low viral load, liver enzymes that were within the high-normal range, and no symptoms of fibrosis or cirrhosis.

"I answered Zora's most pressing question by assuring her that she had plenty of time to try natural therapies before interferon. I explained that I would like to give her nutritional support and detoxification to neutralize the virus and to minimize inflammation. We would know in a few months if this strategy was working; if not she could still begin interferon therapy at the best possible point—while the viral load was still low."

Diet

First, Dr. Singleton told Zora that her daily glass of wine had to go. So did the animal protein in her diet. Because Zora was so active, she was able to eat more than most women without gaining weight. Unfortunately, much of this excess food intake was chicken, red meat, and simple carbohydrates. Zora would need to adopt a low-carbohydrate diet and to avoid all foods that are high in sugar, including sugary fruits like bananas. "Instead, I drew up a detoxification diet. The new diet was heavy in good-quality vegetable protein. I also recommended she increase her intake of alkaline fruits. I recommended deep-sea fish such as mackerel, salmon, tuna, and bass for the omega-3 oils and for the calcium that would help her maintain her bone density and avoid osteoporosis."

"What about fasting?" asked Zora, explaining that she often fasted in conjunction with prayer when she was sick. "I see my doctor, too," she assured Singleton. "But I know that prayer and fasting help me."

Dr. Singleton explained that she could undertake short juice fasts, mixing water and whole juices with pulp and fiber. "But you must avoid plain-water fasts. They might hinder the detoxification process by dumping too many toxins into the liver at once, overwhelming it."

Exercise

Dr. Singleton told Zora to maintain as much of her rigorous physical schedule as she could, and to consider water aerobics on days when she felt too tired for running and swimming. He also suggested that she add fifteen minutes of weight training to her regimen to strengthen her bones because she was showing early signs of bone loss. If she decided to pursue interferon or ribavirin therapy later, maintaining her bone volume would be important because the drugs can leach calcium from the bones. Beginning weight training now would help.

Supplements

Dr. Singleton recommended antioxidant-rich food-based multivitamins without iron such as Just Once by Rainbow Light to replace those she had been taking. He also told her to throw out the iron pills she had been taking since she had been diagnosed as anemic as a child. Her blood tests now revealed that she had high iron levels that could predispose her to cancer, and iron pills were the last thing she needed. If her iron levels didn't fall, he would consider chelation therapy later on.

In an attempt to reduce Zora's viral load to undetectable levels, Dr. Singleton first gave her a large dose of intravenous vitamin C, then put her on a supplementation regimen that included transfer factor for its antiviral and immune-modulating effects. "The medical literature gives ample evidence that transfer factor has a wonderful effect on reducing viral load. [Liver] enzymes invariably come down, so I use it aggressively." He also prescribed for Zora alpha-lipoic acid, MSN (methyl sulfonyl methane) to fortify her immune system and support collagen production, and grapeseed extract (pycnogenol), all of which reduce liver inflammation. Dr. Singleton also recommended UltraClear, a patented compound that enhances the liver's ability to detoxify toxins and other noxious chemicals. (See Chapter 6 for more details about these supplements.)

Finally, Dr. Singleton added the herbs milk thistle and dandelion to Zora's regimen.

Lifestyle Enhancement

Zora was already doing a lot of things right. She was attending a support-group meeting once a month. She is also a devout Christian, and she had escalated her rituals of prayer and meditation since learning she was ill. Instead of meditation, Singleton suggested that she try guided imagery, and showed her how. "It's like meditation on steroids!" Zora said. Zora had used acupuncture for muscle sprains in the past, and Dr. Singleton suggested she try it again for her flulike hepatitis C symptoms. "It's extremely helpful for the discomfort of inflammation," he told her.

Finally, Dr. Singleton pointed out to Zora that her move to Harlem from Washington State had a lot to do with the upsurge in her symptoms. She was living in an area that had an especially dense concentration of liver-toxic chemicals. Some were unavoidable, such as those in the air from auto and chemical exhausts, which were especially plentiful in Harlem. For example, nine of ten toxics-spewing New York City bus depots are located in Harlem. Zora worked out of a home office, so she was constantly exposed. Unless she had a compelling reason for living in the city, Dr. Singleton suggested that Zora consider moving to the suburbs.

Zora's Progress

Zora returned to Dr. Singleton's office every two weeks for monitoring tests. After the first few weeks of her new diet and supplementation regimen, Zora's flulike symptoms—the muscle aches and intermittent fever—began to disappear. A month later, she was able to give up water aerobics for her old swimming-and-running schedule. That same week, she moved from her Harlem apartment to a bedroom community in Westchester with clean air and good water and without New York's witches' brew of liver toxins.

Just six weeks after her first visit to Dr. Singleton, all of Zora's liver enzyme tests had fallen from the high end to the low end of the normal scale. Four months after that, her fatigue had disappeared. "I feel like my old self again," Zora said. "In fact, I'm in training for the New York marathon."

You now know a great deal about hepatitis C, including the many ways you can protect yourself against its ravages. But as was stated in the beginning of this chapter, there is more to learn. Hepatitis C is a relatively "young" diagnosis, and there are many exciting research vistas. We are constantly learning more about which treatments, conventional and complementary, work well. If these patients' successes inspire you to find the treatment plan that works for you, they will have served their purpose.

The next chapter describes treatments for the minority of people with hepatitis C who develop severe cirrhosis or liver cancer. Their livers are so badly injured that they need a liver transplant, and Chapter 10 offers a road map for the journey back from end-stage liver disease.

CHAPTER TEN

Extreme Remedies: Liver Transplants and Experimental Treatment for Advanced Disease

For extreme diseases, employ extreme remedies.
—*Hippocrates*

"You've got a visitor, Mom. From your support group."

I was annoyed when I heard this. I had told my daughter Sarah that I didn't want to see anyone. I sat up in bed, and immediately felt a wave of fatigue wash over me. I tried to look more alert than I felt and hoped my red-rimmed eyes wouldn't give me away. I'd been crying. I had found out a week earlier that my cirrhosis was endstage, and I had sent a message to the support group not to expect me for a while. *Maybe not ever,* I thought. I was on the transplant list, but it was impossible to imagine ever being really well again.

In stepped Anne, with her brown mane bouncing and her skin glowing from a recent vacation in St. Croix. She was wearing a designer pantsuit and a one-hundred-watt smile, and she carried a huge photo album under her arm. I slipped a little lower in the bed, self-conscious about my swollen belly, sallow skin, thinning hair, and wasted frame.

"I want to show you some photographs," she said.

"Sure," I said flatly. I didn't have the energy to feign interest. Didn't she realize that I couldn't care less about her vacation shots? And frankly, we didn't even know each other very well: I was surprised that she had come to my house.

For the next few minutes, Anne showed me photo after photo of herself hollow-eyed, balding, tethered to IV poles, and looking sicker, skinnier, and grayer than I did.

"That was just a year ago!" Anne crowed. "A liver transplant gave me my life back. It will do the same for you."

I owe Anne a great debt. Now I feel that I am going to live. Not survive. Live.

Nancy

Even with the assistance of conventional and alternative medicine, about 15 percent of people with chronic hepatitis C develop either cirrhosis that progresses beyond the liver's ability to recover or liver cancer. The calculated percentages vary from year to year and even within different medical studies, but approximately 10 percent of people with chronic hepatitis C develop endstage cirrhosis and 5 percent develop liver cancer. One to 2 percent develop both.

This is a medical emergency. A functioning liver is essential to the body's major biological processes, and when the liver can no longer carry out any of these functions, a person is said to be in liver failure. A person in liver failure needs immediate liver transplantation. People with endstage cirrhosis or liver cancer have livers that still retain some function, but they will soon need a liver transplant in order to live.

If your liver disease progresses to endstage cirrhosis and liver cancer, practitioners of alternative medicine agree that the time has come to embrace the more vigorous extreme remedies offered by conventional medicine. Even if you have relied upon some combination of conventional, nutritional, herbal, homeopathic, and other complementary approaches up to now, it's time to bring out the big guns.

Transplantation is the removal of a diseased liver and its replacement with a donated, healthier liver. Thomas Starzl performed the first liver transplant at the University of Colorado at Denver in 1963. Today, transplantation is standard therapy for people with endstage liver disease. About twenty thousand liver transplants have been performed at over one hundred U.S. centers, according to United Network for Organ Sharing (UNOS), the national voluntary network that organizes the distribution of transplanted organs. Liver disease caused by hepatitis C is the most common reason for liver transplantation in this country.

As Anne's case demonstrates, liver transplantation works. Three of every four people who receive a new liver are alive five years later, but that statistic doesn't capture the excitement of liver transplantation. Liver transplantation is nothing short of a miracle, because it does more than simply save the lives of endstage hepatitis C patients. It gives them back their energy, hope, and lifestyles. It restores health and vibrancy to people who had become desperately ill, weak, and exhausted by their disease.

Unfortunately, there are not enough donated livers to go around: There are only approximately four thousand livers for the more than seven thousand desperately ill patients who need transplantation each year. This means that people must wait for organs. They are assigned to waiting lists that are prioritized by their degree of illness, but many people die while waiting every year. As this chapter will explain, medical and governmental experts are devising strategies to increase the number of transplants that can be performed each year. Until then, more people must choose to donate their livers if the most desperate needs of people with hepatitis C are to be met.

Conditions That Necessitate a Transplant

Endstage Cirrhosis

The symptoms of endstage cirrhosis are debilitating and dramatic. Hepatitis C patients with endstage cirrhosis are the ones we tend to read about in newspaper and magazine articles. The signs and symptoms include:

- exhaustion that makes one unable to work, exercise, or carry out the normal activities of everyday life.
- jaundice.
- dark urine and light stools.
- pinpoint "blood blisters" and spider angiomas, small blood-swollen veins caused by too little prothrombin, the protein that makes blood clot properly.
- constant, intense itching.
- ascites, fluid retention that causes abdominal swelling.
- easy bruising because of portal hypertension and too little prothrombin.
- mental confusion caused by encephalopathy.
- aversion to smoking and alcohol: People who have tried to kick cigarettes or alcohol for years may suddenly find that smoking or drinking are repugnant to them.
- high fever and chills: These symptoms can indicate life-threatening complications, so you should call a doctor immediately if you experience them.
- persistent hormonal problems that cause gynecomastia (breast growth in men), testicular atrophy, and the loss of pubic and underarm hair.
- depression and anxiety caused by the disease and worsened by the inability to exercise, socialize, or take psychotropic medications.
- blood-clotting problems or misshapen, "clubbed" fingertips and nails.
- grayish, "slate-colored" skin caused by too much iron.

Liver Cancer

Liver cancer is the most feared result of an HCV infection. But keep in mind that although people with chronic hepatitis C are at higher risk for liver cancer, only 5 percent actually develop it. These tend to be people who have been infected with HCV for several decades. Other risk factors include having late-stage cirrhosis, being co-infected with hepatitis B, hepatitis A, or HIV, being older than forty, being male, and having a history of alcohol abuse.

People of geneotype 1 and people who have higher blood levels of virus may be at higher risk for developing liver cancer, but no studies have definitively demonstrated this.

Liver cancer is often diagnosed when monitoring blood tests reveal high or sharply increasing levels of a protein called *alpha-fetoprotein*. A level of more than 500 nanograms per milliliter suggests that the person has liver cancer. But *alpha-fetoprotein* levels do not increase in many people who develop cancer, so doctors also use ultrasound, CT scans, and biopsies to make a diagnosis. These tests are described in Chapter 3.

To treat the cancer, your doctor must first establish that the cancerous tumor began within the liver, which is almost always the case with people who have hepatitis C. If the cancer began elsewhere and spread to the liver, then a liver transplant will not cure it. Most experts use ultrasound to determine whether the tumor began in the liver.

Unfortunately, most people with hepatitis C usually have too much cirrhosis to simply remove the cancerous tumor, since there would not be enough functioning liver tissue to keep the person alive. Only one third of the HCV-infected people who have the tumor surgically removed are alive after five years.

Palliative Treatment

Liver transplantation is the only effective long-term treatment for liver cancer in people with hepatitis C. But while you are waiting for an organ, your doctor may try palliative treatments, which are treatments that aim to control, slow, or stop the damage from a disease or to make the person with the disease more comfortable. Doctors may inject ethyl alcohol (also called ethanol), the purified version of the alcohol in wine and spirits, directly into the tumor. This shrinks it temporarily. Ethanol injection is not a cure, but slows the cancer's growth while you wait for a liver. Doctors also use *chemoembolism,* chemically cutting off the tumor's blood supply in order to starve it. Targeted chemotherapy uses the intravenous infusion of anticancer drugs such as lipiodol to hone in on the liver tumor. Targeted chemotherapy may kill a small tumor, but it is not likely to completely eradicate a large tumor. Radiation is also used, bombarding the tumor with microwaves to shrink it or kill it.

A transplant can cure liver cancer, provided it is small and localized. Only livers that have one or two small cancerous tumors are cured by transplants. Larger tumors or more numerous tumors are likely to have spread beyond the liver. So it is vitally important to find liver cancer early, before it has had a chance to spread.

This means that it is very important to appear for all your regular monitoring tests. Then a tumor will be found early and your doctors can use palliative treatments until a liver becomes available.

The Liver Transplant

Most livers come from cadavers and are donated by generous people who have died in accidents or of diseases that didn't compromise the liver. Adult living donors can also sometimes give parts of their livers. Donor livers remain viable for up to twenty-four hours with the proper handling. The donated liver is tested for blood type and for infections, including HIV and HCV.

In people whose hepatitis C has led to severe cirrhosis, 5 percent are cured of HCV by a transplant. In the remaining 95 percent, HCV quickly infects the new liver. But the new infection tends to cause very little trouble. It progresses very slowly, and never seriously harms the new liver in 80 percent of transplanted people. HCV is still present, but the crippling cirrhosis is gone and usually stays gone. Deathly ill people like Nancy regain their vitality and their liver function.

SIZE DOESN'T MATTER—MUCH. Ideally, the new liver should be the right size for your body, but you can also thrive after receiving one that is too large or too small. If it is too small, it will grow to the appropriate size within weeks. If it is too large, your main concern probably will be cosmetic, because your new liver may visibly bulge under your leotards or bathing suit—a small price to pay to be able to work out and swim again!

TWO LIVERS FROM ONE. You may also receive part of a liver from a living donor. Parents have been donating parts of their livers to their sick children since the late 1980s with good results. The procedure is increasingly being used for adults, too. Living liver donors give part of their healthy liver to a person who needs a transplant. Thanks to the liver's amazing regenerative powers, each has a fully functional complete liver within weeks.

There are too few transplantable livers available, which makes getting a transplant difficult. A recent policy change addresses this liver scarcity. It will encourage hospitals to split all suitable donated livers so that two people—one adult and one child—can receive a transplant from each liver. The new UNOS policy stipulates that any hospital that agrees to split all medically suitable livers will be part of the group that gets the first chance at other donated split livers.

HCV-INFECTED LIVERS. If you are endstage and there are no uninfected livers available, doctors may transplant a liver infected with HCV into you. If an HCV-infected liver is still relatively healthy, without appreciable fibrosis or cirrhosis, this is a good bargain. There is a 15 percent chance that the liver may have belonged to someone who cleared the virus and harbors only antibodies which will not make you ill. But even if the liver is actively infected with HCV, the long life cycle of the disease means that you can live many healthy years with the new liver.

THE TRANSPLANT PROCEDURE. This complicated day-long operation is performed under general anesthesia. First, your own liver is removed in an intricate, lengthy process. The surgeon carefully peels away internal structures in your abdomen to expose your liver. Then she clamps the blood vessels that connect your liver to the rest of your internal organs. Finally, she cuts these blood vessels and removes the diseased liver. She infuses your body with blood-clotting proteins that are normally provided by the liver as well as several pints of blood to replace what you have lost. During the procedure, you can receive as many as twenty pints of blood.

Next, the new liver is sutured to the arteries and veins. The clamps are removed and bile immediately begins to flow from the liver. At this moment, a person who may have had hours or days to live can suddenly look forward to decades of life.

After a few days in the recovery room and intensive care unit, you will be moved to a medical or surgical floor of the hospital for a few weeks while your body adjusts to your new liver. While you are still in the hospital, the hepatitis C virus that remains in your body will probably begin to infect your liver. You will not sense this, so sticking to your regimen of monitoring tests is important even after you have left the hospital.

But the improvement is instantaneous. People who were too weak to move from their beds find that their profound fatigue, pain, and itching disappear. Energy and a normal skin color are immediately restored to their jaundiced, wasted bodies.

The largest risk of liver transplantation is the threat of organ rejection. This occurs when your immune system recognizes a transplanted organ as foreign tissue and responds by attacking your new organ. The most dangerous period is the twenty-four hours immediately after the operation, and the risk of rejection remains high during the month after the transplant. To prevent organ rejection, you will take immunosuppressive drugs such as cyclosporin and cortisone for the rest of your life. These drugs work by crippling the immune system so that it will not recognize and attack the new liver. But they increase your risk of some other illnesses such as cancer and other infectious diseases, which might now proceed, only feebly challenged by the weakened immune system.

Organ rejection is not an all-or-nothing phenomenon: It spans a continuum from mild to severe. You will need a frequent battery of blood tests, liver enzyme tests, and biopsies to make sure that your liver is not exhibiting signs of rejection. The signs of organ rejection include an elevation of liver enzymes such as AST, and higher bilirubin levels. If organ rejection becomes severe, fatigue, loss of appetite, nausea, and even fever may develop. If the initial signs of organ rejection appear, you will be given higher doses of immunosuppressant drugs. These drugs usually arrest the rejection process.

Doses of these drugs, which include steroids, must be carefully adjusted over time. Too-high blood levels of immunosuppressant drugs can cause side effects such as kidney disease and high blood pressure. They can also cause complications such as steroid-induced diabetes, so you will have to learn to monitor your blood glucose, your blood pressure, and other vital signs. Steroids increase your appetite, so you will need to learn new eating strategies. The drugs can also worsen or encourage osteoporosis and fluid retention, but frequent monitoring and dosage adjustments can banish these symptoms.

After the first month, the risk of organ rejection begins to fall and you can take lower doses of antirejection drugs. Half a year after your transplant, your drug dosages will be scaled back even further. You will always need these immunosuppressant drugs, but the gradually lower doses you take will reduce your risks of side effects and other illnesses. Six months after your transplant, you will be back to your normal, pre-illness level of activity. You can work, exercise, play, run, travel—everything a healthy person can do.

Except take a drink. It is common sense that you should avoid anything that taxes your liver. Avoid smoking, coffee, unnecessary medications, and industrial chemicals, too. Eat organic foods and stick with the vegetable-based low-fat diet described in Chapter 9, "Putting It All Together." Avoid shellfish, which can harbor microbes that target the liver. You will also be given a list of liver-toxic drugs to avoid, such as dilantin, birth-control pills, phenobarbital, and hormone replacement therapy.

You're probably wondering how long you can expect to live

with your new liver. Unfortunately, hepatitis C is a relatively new diagnosis, so no definitive long-term follow-up studies have been completed, and doctors cannot yet answer this question. But the prognosis looks very good. At least a ten-year survival seems to be the norm, and plenty of people are alive twenty-five years after their transplants. Because people tend not to need a transplant until they are at least forty years old, many people with transplants may enjoy a near-normal life span: After a transplant, you are likely to die of something other than hepatitis C.

If you do reject your new liver, you may be able to get a second transplant. But people do not do as well after a second procedure: Only 50 percent survive for at least five years after a second transplant.

A transplant is often as good as a cure, but it is expensive. The average transplant cost $250,000 in 1997. Fortunately, more than 80 percent of private health-insurance companies and 94 percent of Medicaid programs fully cover the costs of a liver transplant.

Transplants also carry a psychological cost. Patients who have a liver transplant tend to experience a high degree of anxiety over the process. A study by Patti Case, R.N., of the Baylor University Medical Center in Dallas, found that the times of the first post-transplant biopsy and the first signs of organ rejection were described by participants as their most anxiety-producing experiences of their entire lives.

Fortunately, the end result—a restoration of your health and energy—is well worth it.

Transplant Eligibility

You should understand how doctors decide when you become eligible for a place on the liver-transplantation waiting list. You want to be placed on the waiting list as soon as possible, so it is to your advantage to undergo frequent monitoring of your condition to catch changes in your liver function.

THE CIRRHOSIS POINT SYSTEM.   If you have severe (stage IV) cirrhosis and need a transplant, you must meet certain criteria for eligibility: You must have encephalopathy, bleeding from esophageal varices, ascites, edema, albumin levels that have fallen below 2.5 milligrams per deciliter, or a prothrombin time that has increased at least 3 seconds above the normal time. To evaluate which patients with cirrhosis should be considered for the scarce livers available, transplant centers employ a "point system," which changes from time to time as more or fewer organs become available. This point system includes most of the signs and symptoms of cirrhosis or liver failure.

As you can see on the table below, different intensities of each sign or symptom are assigned different numerical scores, or points, ranging from 1 to 3. As this book went to press, one needed to acquire 7 points to be placed on the waiting list. For example, a person with severe ascites, slight encephalopathy, and a prothrombin time that is 4 seconds longer than normal would earn 7 points and be eligible for a transplant.

Cirrhosis Classification

Sign or symptom	Number of "points"		
	1	**2**	**3**
Ascites	none	slight	moderate/severe
Encephalopathy	none	slight/moderate	moderate/severe
Bilirubin (mg/dl)	less than 2	2–3	greater than 3.0
Albumin (mg/dl)	greater than 3.5	2.8–3.5	less than 2.8
Extension of prothrombin time	1–3 seconds	4–6 seconds	more than 8 seconds

Courtesy Lennox Jeffers, M.D., FACP, the Center for Liver Diseases, University of Miami School of Medicine

TRANSPLANT ELIGIBILITY FOR CANCER PATIENTS. A person who develops liver cancer is typically considered a candidate for liver transplant and put near the top of the list. But here, too, various criteria determine who is eligible. The cancer must be small and localized, and it must not have invaded the portal vein, the major blood vessel that supplies the liver. If there is only one small tumor or three tumors that are less than 3 centimeters (1.2 inches) each, that patient is eligible for a transplant. People with large tumors or many tumors are not considered for transplant, because transplants tend not to cure their cancers. Once on the list, you must be must be screened frequently to make sure the tumor has not grown. Your doctor will discourage tumor growth with ethanol injections, radiation, or chemoembolization, which have been described on page 226.

Who Gets a Liver?

In general, once you are on the waiting list, your chances for a new liver are based on how sick you become. Until recently, your chances of getting an organ were better if the person who donated the organ lived in your area. But the Clinton administration has been urging UNOS to send scarce organs to the sickest patients first, rather than favoring patients who live in the donor's area. In response, UNOS recently adopted a policy that livers are to go to sickest patients first. So if you are given a week or less to live, you are placed at the top of the list. The sickest people are given this priority even if they have already received a liver transplant and are suffering organ rejection. Some feel this policy is unfair because someone who has already been transplanted has priority over people who have yet to receive a liver.

Conditions That Can Compromise Your Ability to Get a Transplant

Whether you have cirrhosis or liver cancer, certain conditions reduce the likelihood that a transplant will cure you, so you will probably not be considered if:

- **You have a current or recent alcohol or drug problem:** The rationale for this policy is that relapse rates for substance abusers are high. But if you have been in recovery for a long time, or your recovery otherwise seems stable, a past substance-abuse problem will not bar you from a transplant.
- **You have certain types of adhesions or complications from prior abdominal surgery.** Replacing your liver is complicated, delicate surgery, and preexisting scar tissue, or adhesions, may make transplant surgery difficult or impossible.
- **You have little or no social support.** Homeless people or people who are estranged from their families are less likely to be placed on the waiting list because they will need help in the difficult months before and after they are transplanted. Experts say that no one can survive the transplant process without people upon whom they can rely to help in caring for them, monitoring their health for danger signs, and providing psychological support.

Liver-Transplant Inequities

Some factors that bar people from liver transplants are not medically based and are not fair. Despite the best efforts of groups such as UNOS and hospital transplant centers, there are some inherently unfair aspects of organ allocation.

A March 1999 Johns Hopkins study determined that gender and ethnicity help determine the medical fates of people who need liver transplants. Ann Klassen, M.D., of the Johns Hopkins School of Public Health, examined UNOS liver waiting lists between 1990 and 1993 and found that "African Americans and Asian Americans were more likely to die waiting than were Caucasians." The report also found that "women, Hispanics, and Asian Americans wait longer than white men" for liver transplants.

It is also an open secret that money and celebrity can tip the scales in a recipient's favor. For example, Mickey Mantle was able to procure a second liver transplant despite a history of alcohol abuse that would normally have rendered a cirrhotic patient ineligible. Pennsylvania governor Robert Casey received a transplant very quickly, although he was less ill than others who had been on the waiting list for weeks or months. Some transplant centers have been accused of making money by pandering to wealthy foreign dignitaries, giving them transplants in exchange for large bequests, while poorer Americans went without the organs they needed.

But the celebrity factor affects the distribution of relatively few organs. The scarcity of donated organs is a much bigger problem. When more people donate livers, fewer people will die of advanced liver disease.

EIGHT WAYS TO MAXIMIZE YOUR CHANCES FOR A TRANSPLANT

You can take steps to improve your chances of receiving a liver:

1. **See your doctor regularly.** How often you see your gastroenterologist for tests and scans will depend upon the nature of your complications. But be sure to keep all your appointments. If you have liver cancer, you must be sure the cancer doesn't grow too large for a transplant, and regular scans will ensure that this is not happening. They will enable you to have the tumor shrunk promptly if it does.

   If you have severe cirrhosis, you want to be placed on the list as soon as possible. You should be tested frequently so that you can be added to the list as soon as your condition makes you eligible. If your condition then worsens and your status becomes more urgent, your name will be eligible for higher placement on the list. But all this can happen only if you have your tests on time.

2. **Get psychological care.** People sick enough to need liver transplants suffer a great deal of anxiety and depression. Gaining solace from counseling, prayer, guided imagery, support groups, and psychotherapy is even more important now. You

must take care of yourself emotionally so that you will have the strength to hold on until an organ becomes available to you.

3. **Mobilize your social support.** You read on page 234 that transplant centers consider social support in determining who is the best candidate for an organ. They feel that a person with a family or social network to care for him or her is most likely to handle the complicated medication regimen and recovery period. If you have a spouse or family who will care for you until you are back on your feet, you are very fortunate.

If not, start constructing your own family to get you through the transplant period. Friends, fellow support-group members, and people from your church, synagogue, or mosque "family" will all step up to the plate for you during this medical emergency. So will members of voluntary organizations such as the American SHARE foundation. But you have to ask them.

4. **Select an experienced transplant center.** Some transplant centers are better then others at using organs efficiently to save transplant patients, and survival rates vary widely at the 117 U.S. transplant centers. Just as with choosing a physician, experience is key. Choose a center that performs a *minimum* of twenty liver transplants a year: The more transplants a center performs, the better.

5. **Maintain your health insurance.** It is not unusual for a family's health insurance policy to cost $400 to $800 a month. If you are employed, your company may help with the payments, but studies suggest that many self-employed people are not insured. Even self-employed people who can afford health insurance sometimes let their policies lapse because they think their money is better spent elsewhere. Many people assume that they can always pick health insurance up again later "when I really need it," but if you obtain health insurance after acquiring HCV, an insurance company may balk at paying for this "pre-existing condition." People who have pursued alternative therapies may reason that paying for insurance is a waste of money because it does not yet

cover many alternative procedures. But if you are infected with HCV, you cannot afford to be without health insurance. If you need a transplant and are not absolutely destitute, you may find it very difficult to qualify for a government program such as Medicaid in order to pay for it.

6. **Seek professional help in paying for a transplant.** Eighty percent of health insurance plans and 95 percent of Medicaid plans pay for liver transplants. But some cities and rural areas do not offer financial support to provide livers for people with low incomes. If you are on Medicaid and have been told that your liver transplant or its associated costs may not be covered, you should ask your doctor for a referral to a social worker who can help you explore your options. You may want to consider moving to an area with a more liberal program for people on Medicaid or governmental assistance.

7. **Stay as active as you can.** You may feel too tired to exercise, but walk every day. The more you can do to maintain your overall health, the longer you can survive and the better your chances for an organ.

8. **Continue nutritional treatments.** Malnutrition and wasting (disease-related muscle and tissue loss) are serious problems in endstage disease, but some special nutritional supplements, such as MCT oil, TPGS (a water-soluble form of vitamin E), and the vitamin C injections mentioned in Chapter 6, can mitigate these nutritional problems until your new liver is in place.

Other Extreme Remedies for Hepatitis C

Not everyone wants to or is able to undergo a liver transplant for severe liver disease. Fortunately, there are promising experimental treatment options for seriously ill people with hepatitis C.

Gene Therapy

Gene therapy works on the theory that one can reprogram the body's cells and cure a disease simply by introducing a healthy gene into the body. The healthy gene, or "repair" gene, is carried to the correct site—in this case liver cells—via a *vector*. A vector is an infectious agent such as a virus. The vector directs the liver cell to churn out a therapeutic protein that generates tissues with entirely new, healthy properties. A key concern is to find a virus that won't cause disease and that won't be attacked and nullified by the person's immune system.

There are five gene therapy centers in Europe and ten in the United States: Contact the American Liver Foundation or U.S. Department of Health and Human Services for the site nearest you. Phone numbers for both agencies are given in Chapter 11.

The Artificial Liver

James Kelly, M.D., Ph.D., a biochemist from Houston, Texas, is testing his invention, the Hepatix artificial liver, on English patients with liver failure. The Hepatix works something like an artificial kidney to filter impurities and toxins from the blood, but it is much more complex. The patient's blood is passed through cylinders that contain cartridges of live, cloned human liver cells. These human liver cells provide 20 to 30 percent of the liver's other natural functions. Dr. Kelley has used the machine on five acute-liver-failure patients in London's King's College Hospital. For four of these patients, the Hepatix provided a lifeline that gave their livers time to recover function. These four patients are now healthy, but the fifth patient, who was sicker, died.

The "Inhibition of Translation" Approach

"Translation" is the process by which a virus hijacks cells to make its own proteins and make copies of itself. Researchers are trying to devise a slew of new antiviral agents that will work by "inhibition of translation," or stopping the virus from making proteins and new viruses. There are many specific techniques for attempting this. One example is a process being performed in clinical trials by Chiron Corporation.

If scientists find a way to stop the HCV virus from using liver cells to replicate, this strategy would be as good as a cure, because the immune system could kill the invading viruses and there would be no viral replacements made.

Intravenous Protein Supplements

This experimental liquid may reduce the number of people who die during liver surgery. This supplement containing branched-chain amino acids (which the body uses to make proteins) was given through intravenous tubes to several groups of people undergoing surgery for liver cancer. It may benefit people undergoing transplants and other types of liver surgery as well.

The branched-chain amino acids reduced the number of deaths in people with liver cancer and reduced nearly every important side effect of surgery. People who underwent this therapy had better liver function.

It works because branched-chain amino acids seem to lower the levels of ammonia, a toxic by-product of the body's protein metabolism.

The formulation consists of branched-chain amino acids, dextrose in a fat emulsion. The liquid was administered to patients intravenously during the fourteen-day period immediately before and after surgery for liver cancer. As with any new experimental procedure, unforeseen risks and complications may emerge.

What You Need to Know about Clinical Trials

If you develop severe liver disease, you will hear a lot of buzz about clinical trials. The chief advantage to participating in a test of an experimental treatment, or a clinical trial, is that you could be among the first to reap the benefits of a potential cure. All experimental studies on humans must be approved by the FDA. In addition, they have been approved by a local institutional review board, a group of scientists and community representatives who scrutinize the proposed study. Their job is to ensure that the study is as safe as possible and that volunteers will be fully informed of the nature of the study and of the risks they are undertaking.

But the downside of any experimental trial is risk. There is always the risk, however slight, that a relatively untried treatment will injure or even kill human volunteers.

Just because a trial is willing to enroll you doesn't mean that participating is the best decision for your health. No matter how humane and conscientious he or she is, the doctor who conducts the trial is primarily interested in the experiment. Your doctor, on the other hand, is interested in you and in your health. So be sure to ask your doctor to evaluate any trial that intrigues you before you join it. Obtain printed information from the Web site or the investigators and share it with your doctor so he or she can tell you whether it is safe and appropriate for you.

EXPERIMENTAL-TREATMENT CHECKLIST

1. **Talk to your doctor.** Your doctor can tell you about trials in your area that offer promising treatments for hepatitis C, end-stage cirrhosis, or liver cancer, or that address specific medical problems you are having. She will protect you from any experiments that she thinks are unsafe or inappropriate.

2. **Choose "Phase 3" trials.** People who want to volunteer for medical research can participate in any of three phases of trial tests. Phase 1 trials test for the safety limits of a drug, Phase 2 trials test for efficacy, and Phase 3 trials involve fine-tuning a drug before its market release. Phase 3 trials are the ones you want to seek out, because drugs in these trials have passed safety and effectiveness tests. But there is always some risk involved.

3. **Find a trial that's right for you.** After you have talked to your doctor, you can do some of your own medical detective work. Contact the liver disease center of the university-related medical center that is nearest you. Ask a member of the reference staff in the medical library of your hospital for help.

Consult some of the transplantation advocacy organizations and Web sites listed at the end of this chapter and in Chapter 11. Newspapers carry notices of clinical trials in their health calendar sections. Ask friends in your support group what they have heard and what they have tried.

4. **Guard your legal rights.** No matter what you have signed, you cannot be forced to participate in any tests and you can drop out of an experimental treatment at any time, even if you have been paid to participate. Investigators must inform you of any dangers with a drug or procedure that emerge during the trial.

5. **Ask lots of questions** before agreeing to participate, including: *What are the side effects? Why is the study being done? What is its purpose? What kind of tests and treatments does the study involve? What will happen if I enter the study? What might this treatment do to me? How can the study affect my everyday life? (Will I be nauseous? Irritable? Unable to drive?) How long will the study last? Will I be hospitalized? If so, for how long and how often? If I am injured as a result of the study, what treatment will I receive? Could my name or identifying information be made available to other researchers or agencies?* (You should seek a trial that guarantees confidentiality.) *Do any of the researchers have a financial interest in the product they are testing?* (If so, reconsider joining this trial: A financial interest in the outcome is a real threat to experimental objectivity.)

Hundreds of new clinical trials emerge every day, and every day, old ones stop accepting patients. Thus, it would make little sense to list information about specific clinical trials here, even if there were enough space. Instead the address for CenterWatch, a Web site that maintains information on current clinical trials, is listed at the end of this chapter. Additional sites are listed in Chapter 11, "Healing Resources."

The Next Challenges

The biggest hurdle in devising new treatments for hepatitis C is the difficulty scientists are having in culturing the virus, that is, growing it in the laboratory. Once this challenge is overcome, as it has been for polio, smallpox, and other viruses that once stumped researchers, we can expect better treatments. Culturing HCV in the laboratory will be the first step toward a vaccine and toward finding more effective, less extreme options for people with advanced liver disease from hepatitis C.

Meanwhile, there is something each of us can do. Urge your friends and family to sign their organ donor cards so that every possible liver can be used to restore the lives of people suffering with severe liver disease. In this way, everyone can help to keep the miracles coming.

Perhaps one of the experimental modalities you read about here or in Chapter 4 will prove an even safer, more effective answer. A cure is the ultimate goal of everyone who cares about people with hepatitis C. Until there is a cure, Chapter 11 will help you keep up and continue your hepatitis C education. It offers an extensive list of resources—social, medical informational, and online.

For more information

Organizations
United Network for Organ Sharing (UNOS)
  (804) 330-8500
  The Web site, www.ew3.att.net/unos, offers
  many details on obtaining an organ transplant.
Transplant Recipient International Organization (TRIO)
  1000 16th Street, NW, Suite 602
  Washington, DC 20036-5705
  (800) TRIO-386; (202) 293-0980
  Web site: www.trioweb.org
  National support group for transplant patients and their families

U.S. Department of Health and Human Services
  Division of Transplantation
  5600 Fishers Lane, Room 481
  Rockville, MD 20857
  (301) 443-7577
  Web site: www.hrsa.gov/osp/dot

Online Sources
American SHARE Foundation
  www.asf.orgl
  This extensive transplant-related Web site offers links to other helpful sites.
Hepatitis Haven Web Site
  www.tiac.net/users/birdlady/hep.html
  Offers transplant information, a directory, and copious drug information for people with hepatitis C.
CenterWatch Patient Notification Service
  www.centerwatch.com/PATEMAILhtm
  This site enables you to register for e-mail notifications of every new
  clinical trial investigating hepatitis C. It also alerts you to new HCV
  drugs as they are approved by the FDA.

CHAPTER ELEVEN

Healing Resources

This chapter lists resources that can help you to live well with hepatitis C. These include:

- Books and other publications
- Voluntary organizations
- Governmental agencies
- Resources for patients
- Selected Web sites

WEB SITE WARNING. The Internet can provide useful and accurate information on gastrointestinal diseases, but use care. When Case Western Reserve University researchers reviewed the validity of one hundred sites on major gastrointestinal diseases, including hepatitis C, they questioned the validity of 17.6 percent of the 4.3 million "hits" for hepatitis C. This means that one of every six sites contains questionable advice or unsubstantiated information.

Unless a Web site is sponsored by a university medical center or another well-credentialed medical group, there's a chance that you will encounter some of the misinformation circulating everywhere in cyberspace. The following sites have been carefully selected for interest and accuracy, but because some of them are intended as mutual-support sites, not medical education sites, I do not vouch for the accuracy of the information dispensed by any site or person listed below.

No matter what pearls of information you glean from the Internet or from an organization listed below, remember that your doctor is the final arbiter of what is safe and effective treatment for you: Always run advice by him or her before trying it.

Books

Fleming, Thomas, Ph.D., chief editor. *The PDR for Herbal Medicines,* 1st edition. Medical Economics Co., 1998, $59.95. A clear, exhaustive, extensively illustrated and cross-referenced guide to the pharmacology and uses of herbs.

Fugh-Berman, Adriane, M.D. *Alternative Medicine: What Works.* William & Wilkins, 1997, $14.95. A clear, readable, and wonderfully balanced scientific assessment of alternative approaches to health and disease.

Herbert, Victor, M.D. *Total Nutrition.* St. Martin's Press, 1995, $17.95. This 800-page tome on nutrition is big, well-written, and comprehensive— a bargain. Its 41 chapters are packed with useful basic information in clear language, including hundreds of tables, sample menus, and graphics. But be warned: This book is quite conservative, and you will find no information on alternative nutritional approaches, with which Dr. Herbert displays little patience.

Hobbs, Christopher. *Milk Thistle: The Liver Herb.* Botanica Press, 1984. This 32-page booklet makes a case for milk thistle's role in treating hepatitis. It offers useful information on the herb's traditional uses and recent human studies of the herb.

————. *Foundations of Health: Healing with Herbs and Other Foods.* Botanica Press, 1992, $13.95. This book includes copious information about herbs and foods that are useful in treating hepatitis. But its author relies heavily on anecdotal and historical information and makes some uncritical recommendations. This book will be very useful in conjunction with advice from your physician.

Other Publications

Focus: On Hepatitis
    Quantum Media Group
    130 Prim Road, Suite 510
    Colchester, VT 05446
    (802) 655-2715
    National hepatitis C newsletter

Henkel, John. "Hepatitis C." *FDA Consumer,* March 1, 1999.

Hepatitis C Fact Sheet. www.cdc.gov/ncidod/diseases/hepatitis/c/
    faq.htm

Hepatitis C Questions and Answers, www.cdc.gov/ncidod/diseases/
    hepatitis/c/faq.htm

Hepatitis Education Project, www.halcyon.com/jevo/HEP/. Publishes
    a quarterly newsletter and educational materials.

Hepatitis Weekly, www.holonet.net/homepage/IH.htm. News, research,
    and journal articles on hepatitis.

Progress. A quarterly consumer newsletter published by the American
    Liver Foundation.

Voluntary Organizations

The American Liver Foundation
    1425 Pompano Avenue
    Cedar Grove, NJ 017201
    (800) 223 256-2550; (888) 4-HEPUSA; (973) 256-2550
    A nonprofit health agency that promotes research, education, and
    support groups dedicated to curing hepatitis. Its Web site, http://liver
    foundation.org, offers updates on treatment and research as well as
    frequently asked questions (FAQs) regarding hepatitis C.

Global Hepatitis Support Network
    611 Avenue of the Americas, Suite 148
    New York, NY 10011
    or 130 Prim Road, Suite 511
    Colchester, VT O8446
    (802) 655-2579

This nonprofit organization provides information and support to hepatitis C patients.

The Hepatitis C Foundation

1502 Russett Drive

Warminster, PA 18974

(215) 672-2606

This foundation supports research and development of additional treatments for hepatitis C. Its 24-hour toll-free help line also provides personal support, referrals, and information. The foundation also has a political-action arm that promotes projects that encourage better research funding.

Hepatitis Foundation International

30 Sunrise Terrace

Cedar Grove, NJ 07000

(800) 891-0707 *or* (201) 239-1035

Provides physician referrals, updated treatment information and access to a telecommunications network of patients with similar ailments.

Hepatitis C Latino Organizations

Spanish-language information about hepatitis C.

www.chasque.apc.org/freno/hepcespa.html

Latino Organization for Liver Awareness

(888) 367-5652; (718) 892-8697

Offers bilingual support.

Family Issues

The Well Spouse Foundation

P.O. Box 28876

San Diego, CA 92198

(619) 673-9043; (914) 357-8513

Provides emotional and political support to spouses of the chronically ill; produces a bimonthly newsletter.

HepCan-Kids

Information and help for the parents of children with hepatitis C.

www.findmail.com/group/hepcan-kids/info.html

BACafe

www.flash.net/~twb/BACafe/

Offers a page for kids with HCV as well as other support and information about hepatitis C, Web sites, and information for the newly diagnosed.

Governmental Agencies

Centers for Disease Control and Prevention (CDC)

Hepatitis Branch, Mailstop G37

Division of Viral and Rickettsial Diseases

National Center for Infectious Diseases

Centers for Disease Control and Prevention

Atlanta, GA 30333

CDC Public Inquiries: (800) 311-3435

CDC Hepatitis Hotline: (404) 332-4555. This hotline permits you to automatically request information that will be faxed to your machine.

Departments of Public Health

For information about hepatitis C in your state, call your State Department of Public Health, Epidemiology Division.

The National Institutes for Health (NIH) is the research arm of the Public Health Service, U.S. Department of Health and Human Services. Several of its institutes conduct research on hepatitis viruses, including the National Institute of Allergy and Infectious Diseases (NIAID) and the National Institute of Diabetes and Digestive and Kidney Diseases (NIDDK). The home page for the NIH, www.nih.gov/, points you to information on hepatitis.

U.S. Department of Health and Human Services

Division of Transportation

5600 Fishers Lane, Room 481

Rockville, MD 20857

(301) 443-7577

www.hrsa.sav/osp/dot

NIAID Office of Communications

Building 31

Room 7A50

Bethesda, MD 20892

(301) 496-5717

Press releases, fact sheets, and other materials are available on the Internet via the NIAID home page:www.niaid.nih.gov/.

National Institute of Diabetes and Digestive and Kidney Diseases (NIDDK) Clearinghouse

2 Information Way

Bethesda, MD 20892-3570

Write to this address for a packet of materials on hepatitis C.

Web site: http://niddk.nih.gov/NIDDK_HomePage.html

Selected Web Sites

American Association for the Study of Liver Diseases

http://hepar-sfgh.ucsf.edu/

Offers information on meetings, publications, and courses for liver disease specialists.

The Canadian Liver Foundation

www.liver.ca

Home page of Canada's premier voluntary organization for liver diseases

CDC Emerging Diseases Page

www.cdc.gov/ncidod/EID/eid.htm

Updates on emerging diseases, including hepatitis C

Chronic Hepatitis Answering Page

www.hepatitis_central.com/hcv/drs/askdr.html

Ask your HCV questions of expert physicians.

Columbia University Diseases of the Liver

http://cpmcnet.columbia.edu/dept/gi/references.html

The university's hepatology site offers lots of information about liver diseases. A related site, **Current Papers on Liver Disease,** offers even more:

http://cpmcnet.columbia.edu/dept/gi/references.html

http://koop.dartmouth.edu, accessible via American Online and Disney's GOnetwork. This is an older site at Dartmouth University that offers good but dated basic science information about managing hepatitis C; its inspiring "personal stories" section is up-to-date.

National Digestive Diseases Information Clearinghouse

www.nddk.nih.gov

(301) 654-3810

Provides facts on hepatitis C.

Hepatitis C Society

http://web.idirect.com/-hepc/

Home page for the Hepatitis C Society in Canada with information about HCV

HEP Education Project

www.scn.org/health/hepatitis/

Nonprofit corporation providing education, materials, and information about support groups.

Hepatitis WebRing

www13.pair.com/jude/hepring

also: www.alusa.com/fineart/em.hepc.html

Home page for the Hepatitis WebRing, dedicated to providing a simple yet exciting and efficient means of locating Web sites with information pertaining to hepatitis.

Hep C Connection

www.hepc-connection.org

Helpful site with lots of information about hepatitis C

Hepatitis A, B, and C: Questions and Answers

gopher:www.gopher.uiuc.edu/oo/UI/CSF/health/heainfo/diseases/contag/hepa

A brief page describing the differences between various types of hepatitis, with information on prevention and treatment.

Patient Information and Advocacy

www.patientsamerica.com

This comprehensive site was founded by Dr. Steven J. Bock, who has also established the Rhinebeck Health Center in upstate New York and the Center for Progressive Medicine in Albany. It offers information on progressive medicine as well as assistance in locating medical care.

Mutual Support

HCV Support and Info

http://members.aol.com/hcv30204s8/Index.html

A wealth of links, chat rooms, personal stories, and local support groups

Hepatitis Mutual Support

http://members.aol.com/VikkiSM/hepage.html/

Links to many informational sites on hepatitis, as well as mutual support

Hep C Forum Mailing List

A mailing list for patients with hepatitis C. To subscribe, send an e-mail message to majordomo@lists.vossnet.co.uk and type SUB-SCRIBE HEPC in the body of the message. Or visit the forum's Web site at: http://village.vosnet.co.uk/c/crina/maillist.htm

Hepatitis Newsgroup

USENET sci.med.diseases.hepatitis

A lively newsgroup for sharing information, research news, and experiences

HEPV-L

Patients with chronic hepatitis C share advice, tips, and personal stories on this mailing list. To subscribe, type the words SUBSCRIBE HEPV-L <YOUR FULL NAME> in the body of the e-mail message. Send the message to: listserv@sjuvm.stjohns.edu.

Finding a Health-Care Professional

Hepatitis C Foundation

www.hepcfoundation.org

E-mail: hepatitis_c_foundation@msn.com

Information, personal support, and referrals

Hepatitis Foundation International

http://cpmcnet.columbia.edu/dept/gi/hcpint.html

Resources, information updates, support, and links to books and other products

Hepatitis C Chat Rooms

Land of Waz Hepatitis
www.asan.com/users/wazzie/wizpagez.htm
Hepatitis site with a Java-enabled health chat box

Priority Healthcare Corporation of Altamonte Springs, Florida, hosts
seven chat rooms at www.hepatitisneighborhood.com/

Conventional Treatment Information

Hepatitis and Liver Disease Referral Network
www.arens.com/hepnet/
This site offers a list of prominent hepatologists.

Ribavirin
www.aidsinfonyc.org/pwahg/info/riba.html, and www.hep.help.com
This home page for Schering-Plough, the makers of interferon, offers information about its combination drug ribavirin, which is described in Chapter 4.

CenterWatch Clinical Trials Listing Service
www.centerwatch.com/PATEMAIL.htm
This site is for people with hepatitis C who want information about
clinical trials and new FDA-approved drugs. A related site, www.
centerwatch.com, enables you to sign up for e-mail notifications of
every new clinical trial that is being investigated for action against
hepatitis C.

Subscriptions to *Ironic Blood,* which deals with iron levels and
hepatitis, a topic covered in Chapters 4, 5, and 6, are available
through the IOD Association office at (561) 840-8512. Or write:

IOD Association
433 Westwind Drive
North Palm Beach, FL 33408
Ironic Blood is also available via e-mail: iod@emi.net

Healthcare Abroad
243 Church Street West
Vienna, VA 22180
(800) 237-6615
(703) 281-9500

Information on how to minimize the risk of contracting HCV while traveling

The International Association for Medical Assistance to Travellers
417 Center Street
Lewiston, NY 14092
(716) 754-4883
Information on how to minimize the risk of contracting HCV while traveling

International SOS Assistance
P.O. Box 11568
Philadelphia, PA 19116
Within PA: (215) 244-1500
Outside PA: (800) 523-8930
Information on how to minimize the risk of contracting HCV while traveling

Complementary Treatment

The American Holistic Medical Association
6728 Old McClean Village Drive
McClean, VA 22101
(703) 556-9728
Fax: (703) 556-8729
E-mail: ahma@degnon.org
You can access the AHMA personal physician referral directory for free online at www.holisticmedicine.org. This is a list of licensed physicians who have trained in a variety of complementary approaches. Or you can mail $10 with a request for a hard copy of the list.

Andrew Weil, M.D.
Director
Program in Integrative Medicine
University of Arizona School of Medicine
P.O. Box 5099
Tucson, AZ 85724-5099
(520) 626-5077
Fax: (520) 626-2757

The related Weil Institute trains primary-care physicians in integrative medical approaches. Patients are treated by the group. If you live in or can take a sojourn to the Tucson area, you may wish to apply for treatment.

Transplantation

United Network for Organ Sharing (UNOS)
1100 Boulders Parkway, Suite 500
P.O. Box 13770
Richmond, VA 23225-8770
(804) 330-8500
The Web site, www.unos.org/frame_default.asp, offers many details on obtaining an organ transplant.

Transplant Recipient International Organization (TRIO)
National support group for transplant patients and families
1000 16th Street, NW, Suite 602
Washington, DC 20036-5705
(800) TRIO-386
(202) 293-0980
Web site: www.trioweb.org

Transplant Recipient International Organization (TRIO)
Nationwide support group for patients and families
1735 I Street, NW, Suite 317
Washington, DC 20036-5705
(800) TRIO-386
(202) 293-0980
Web site: www.trioweb.org

American Share Foundation
www.asf.org
A large transplant-related Web site, with links to other helpful sites

Hepatitis Haven
www.tiac.net/users/birdlady/hep.html
A Web site offering a directory, links, transplant information, and drug information resources for people with HCV

U.S. Department of Health and Human Services
Division of Transplantation

5600 Fishers Lane, Room 481
Rockville, MD 20857
(301) 443-7577
Web site: www./origville.edu/library/ekstrom/govpubs/federal/
agencies/bhs/transdic.html

Columbia-Presbyterian Department of Surgery
622 West 168th Street, PH-14 Stemm
New York, NY 10032
(877) 548-3763 (877-LIVER MD), toll-free
Referral Hotline, 24 hours, 7 days: (800) 543-2782
Referrals by fax: (212) 305-4343
To e-mail the program directors:
Jean C. Emond, M.D., Surgical Director: je111@columbia.edu
Robert S. Brown, Jr., M.D., Medical Director: rb464@columbia.edu

Political Activism

Hep-C ALERT!
www.hep-C-alert.org
Nonprofit activist organization

HCVActivist Mailing List
This list is concerned with letter writing, political action, and reform
in connection with hepatitis C research and funding. To subscribe,
type SUBSCRIBE HCV ACTIVIST in the body of the e-mail message and send the message to: majordomo@statsrus.com.

Drug Treatment Resources

Cocaine Anonymous
3740 Overland Avenue, Suite G
Los Angeles, CA 90034
(800) 347-8998
Provides information on cocaine addiction and rehabilitation programs.

Drug Abuse Information and Treatment Referral Line
National Institute on Drug Abuse
11426 Rockville Pike, Suite 410
Rockville, MD 20852
(800) 662-4357; Spanish, (800) 662-9832; hearing impaired,

(800) 228-0427, 9:00 A.M. to 3:00 A.M. (eastern time) Monday–Friday, noon to 3:00 A.M. (eastern time) Saturday and Sunday. Provides counseling and referral services to callers. Also provides general information on substance abuse and addiction.

Families Anonymous

P.O. Box 528

Van Nuys, CA 91408

(800) 736-9805; (818) 989-7841

Provides information for families with children who have substance abuse or behavioral problems. Also provides counseling for family members and friends.

National Clearinghouse for Alcohol and Drug Information

6000 Executive Boulevard, Suite 402

Rockville, MD 20852

(800) 729-6686

Provides information and referrals to callers with questions about alcohol- and drug-treatment programs.

National Cocaine Hotline

P.O. Box 100

Summit, NJ 07901-0100

(800) 262-2463

Provides information and referrals to drug-treatment and rehabilitation programs. Also answers specific questions on drug abuse.

ABOUT THE AUTHORS

Harriet A. Washington is a science and medical writer who has won some of the most prestigious awards in journalism. She spent seven years as a newspaper editor at several metropolitan dailies, including *USA Today*. She has won the Harvard Journalism Fellowship for Advanced Studies in Public Health, a John S. Knight Fellowship at Stanford University, and fellowships from the Council for the Advancement of Science Writing and the Stanford Professional Publishing Course.

Ms. Washington has been a teaching assistant at the Harvard School of Public Health and an adjunct professor at the Rochester Institute of Technology. She has taught at branches of the State University of New York and Writers&Books as well.

She has been contributing editor of *Heart & Soul* magazine and medical columnist for *Emerge* magazine, and has published in such venues as the *Harvard Health Letter, Health, Essence,* and *Psychology Today*. Her medical investigative awards include the NABJ First Prize for her series "Health Care Reform" and two first-place Unity awards. In 1999, her work won the Congressional Black Caucus's Beacon of Light award.

Ms. Washington's work has appeared in academic publications as well, among them the *New England Journal of Medicine, Nature,* the *Harvard Public Health Review,* and the *Harvard AIDS Review*. She is founding editor of the *Harvard Journal of Minority Public Health* and co-author of *Health and Healing for African Americans*.

She lives in New York City with her husband, Ron DeBose, a screenwriter.

Steven J. Bock, M.D., the author of the Foreword, received his medical degree from New York Medical College in 1971. His practice integrates his expertise in complementary and traditional medicine. He is the co-author with his brother Dr. Kenneth Bock of *Natural Relief for Your Child's Asthma* (HarperPerennial, 1999). They have jointly founded two health centers in upstate New York: the Rhinebeck Health Center and the Center for Progressive Medicine in Albany.